STRAIGHT FROM THE
HORSE'S MOUTH

STRAIGHT FROM THE HORSE'S MOUTH

CHERYL GREEN & FAITH HANCOCK

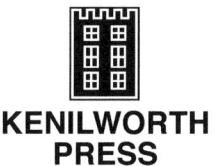

KENILWORTH PRESS

First published 2025

Kenilworth Press
An imprint of Quiller Publishing
The Hill, Stroud
Gloucestershire, GL5 4EP

www.quillerpublishing.com

Copyright © Cheryl Green & Faith Hancock, 2025

The right of Cheryl Green & Faith Hancock to be identified as the Authors of this work has been asserted in accordance with the Copyright, Designs and Patents Act 1988.

ISBN 978 1 9100 1667 1 (paperback)
ISBN 978 1 9100 1668 8 (ebook)

All rights reserved. No part of this book may be reprinted or reproduced or utilised in any form or by any electronic, mechanical or other means, now known or hereafter invented, including photocopying and recording, or in any information storage or retrieval system, without the permission in writing from the Publishers.
Disclaimer of Liability
The information contained in this book is true and complete to the best of our knowledge. All recommendations are made without any guarantee on the part of the publisher and authors, who also disclaim any liability incurred in connection with the use of this data or specific details. The opinions expressed by the authors in this book are their own views and may or may not be the views of others.

Kenilworth Press encourages the use of approved safety helmets in all equestrian sports and activities.

British Library Cataloguing in Publication Data.
A catalogue record for this book is available from the British Library.

1 2 3 4 5 6 7 8 9 10

Typesetting by SJmagic DESIGN SERVICES, India.
Printed in the UK.

Appointed GPSR EU Representative: Easy Access System Europe Oü, 16879218
Address: Mustamäe tee 50, 10621, Tallinn, Estonia
Contact Details: gpsr.requests@easproject.com, +358 40 500 3575

CONTENTS

1	About Me	7
2	Learning to Listen	12
3	Ranger	19
4	Bodyworkers	26
5	Gut Feelings	39
6	Feet	57
7	On the Tracks	64
8	Behavioural Issues	73
9	What to Wear	81
10	Oils	87
11	Case Studies	95
12	People Hearing Without Listening	180
13	Frequently Asked Questions	184

Acknowledgements	188
Index	190

I

ABOUT ME

If you're like a lot of people, you are probably thinking that anyone who says they can communicate with animals is a little bit bonkers. You might snigger behind your hand and imagine someone who is like a cross between Mystic Meg and Steve Irwin. I know what you're thinking – surely anyone who claims to be able to hear what an animal is saying is definitely weird. Perhaps they waft about in flowing robes, trail incense behind them like a smokescreen and talk in hushed tones about their 'gift'. Then they'll charge you extortionate amounts to hear what your horse is saying and sweep off into the sunset, leaving you none the wiser and a great deal more cynical! This could not be further from the truth for me.

I am just about as down to earth a person as you could ever wish to meet. There's no ceremony, no wafting incense, no chanting – I just listen to your horse, then tell you what they are saying to me. It's the most incredibly rewarding job in the world, because of how much of a difference I can make to the horse and the owner.

I don't know how I do what I do – I am just able to do it. Of course, I get a fair amount of scepticism, from my friends and family – and even from myself. I often tell new clients, 'I only have to convince *you* once that I'm the real deal; I have to convince *myself* every damn day!'

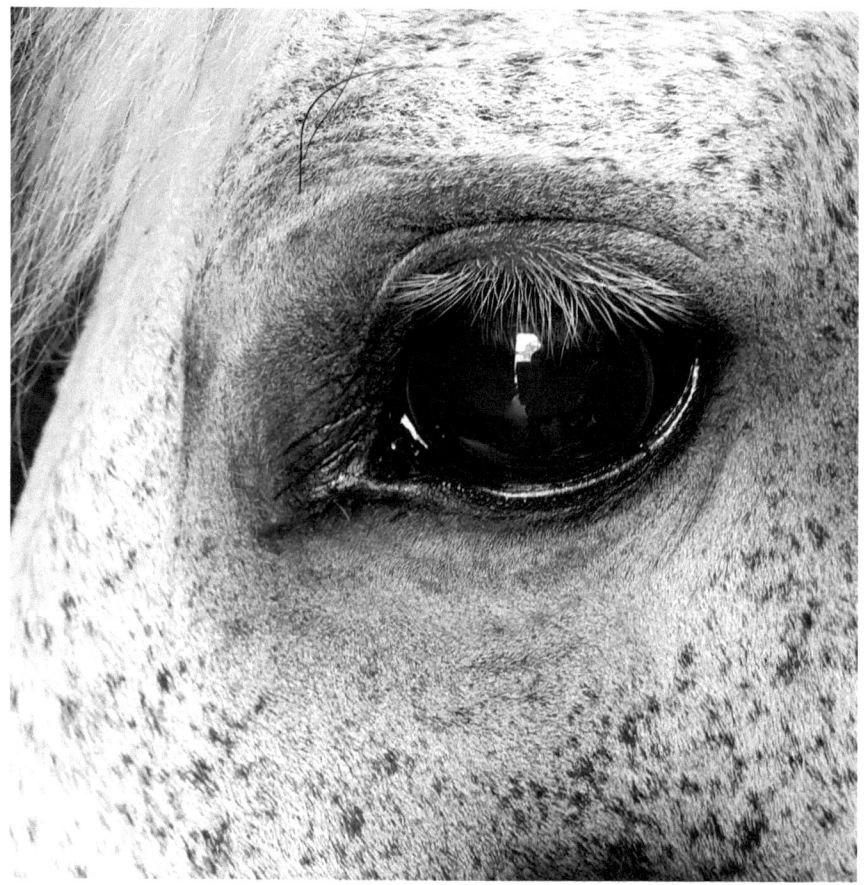

The eyes are the window to the soul. (Tayah Birkett)

Put quite simply, I am an equine communicator – I can hear what horses are trying to communicate and I use this to help their owners to understand them better, and to improve the lives of both the horses and the people who love them. There is so much more that we can do with our horses once we understand what it is that they need, or how they are feeling – just like people, really.

I didn't set out to be an equine communicator, it came to me, as so many things do in life that are right. I firmly believe that I was called to do this; it is and always has been my purpose in life – despite a few false starts and time spent in jobs that I hated or were not fulfilling. I wonder how many of us are now doing a job that we never thought we would be doing when we were younger?

When I started out, it was a sideline and a hobby; I was working in the financial industry, which was, as you can imagine, a far cry from talking to horses! I have always been interested in the alternative side of life and I was practising Tarot and doing readings for my friends. It then just snowballed over time. I told a few friends what their horses were saying, they told their friends, who then told *their* friends, and pretty soon I had to quit my bank job as I was taking on many more horse clients.

When I began, I would drive all around the countryside visiting yards and stables, but as my client base has increased so dramatically, I now mostly tend to work from a photograph of the horse's eye. The eyes are the window to the soul and I can get all the initial information I need from tapping into the horse through this photograph. I bet this makes you even more disbelieving, right? How can I talk to horses at all, let alone without even meeting them in person? Again, there's no way of explaining this. It is what it is, and I know because of my testimonials that I am accurate in what I see and hear, despite not always meeting the horses and owners I work with in person.

There are no weird rituals, chanting, or anything remotely 'way-out' about what I do – I just listen, and the horses talk. I cannot explain the scientific process of this probably because science, although it is wonderful in so many ways, has no explanation for it. We'll have a chat a bit later about how you can do this with your horse, too, and no, you don't need fancy robes or a crystal ball to do so. Yes, you might feel a bit silly the first time you do it, but I promise you it's just the same as saying 'good morning' to your partner, chatting to the kids, or catching up with a friend.

I was prodded in the direction of communicating with horses by my own heart horse Ranger, who was – and is – my inspiration, guide and teacher. I miss him every single day, but he is always with me in spirit. More about him later, too, because he demanded and deserves his very own chapter.

Possibly because of my relationship with Ranger, I specialise in those horses that have been considered 'nasty', 'dangerous', 'untrainable', or 'should be shot' – and I have managed to save many of these horses from being destroyed, simply by listening and learning what their problems are, then helping their owners work through them. Often people come to me after having exhausted every other lead to see what is 'wrong' with their horse, and I have had many encounters with people who were incredibly sceptical, but then they have come around to a more open-minded point of view, having heard what their horses, through me, are saying.

It's really hard, isn't it, when you've had the vet out countless times; fixed the tack; had the feet done; checked the teeth are fine; ensured the diet is perfect; played matchmaker with the herd and seen that best friends are together; the accommodation is ideal – and yet your horse still has problems. Well, it's not too far out of this world to suggest that there might be something deeper going on and that being able to find out what your horse actually thinks and feels might be an answer to the problem.

This is where I come in. I often work with various horse bodyworkers – mainly Bowen therapists, but also others, too, which is a very interesting experience, especially if we are able to simultaneously communicate with and treat the horse. Many of my favourite bodyworkers have started out very sceptical (and some tell me they still are, and are always trying to catch me out!) until they start the horse on their treatments and realise that the problems the horse has told me about are right there in their bodies, despite not having been obvious from the outside.

I am not someone who pretends to understand how I do what I do – all I know is that I do it. I can 'hear' horses speaking to me, as if they were having a conversation like you and me. Why do

About Me

I do it? Well, there is no other path I would rather be on. I count my blessings every day that I am lucky enough to do a job that I love so much and one that has made such a difference to so many horses and their people.

I live a quiet and happy life with my beloved family – my husband, who was my childhood sweetheart, and our beautiful twins. We have a Devon Rex cat and a pointer dog, both rescued from Cyprus. I did own an ex-racehorse after Ranger, then a cheeky Welsh Section D, but because of circumstances I have not had any other horses. I just don't have enough time these days. I often come across horses that I feel would be the perfect fit – but having had the incredible relationships with all my horses, I don't feel the urge to get another one of my own at this time. Besides, doing this job, I get my horsey fix all day, every day!

I love what I do. It's so interesting and no two days are ever the same. Some horses are incredibly funny; some are in pain; some are crying out for help; some are simply happy and content. If I can help a single horse and owner in a day, I can go to bed happy. I am determined to improve life for horses and their people, and I am dedicated to changing the world, one horse at a time.

2

LEARNING TO LISTEN

I was born into a military family and animals have been a big feature of my life for as long as I can remember. We had rescue animals all through my growing-up years – many of whom had been badly treated and came from awful surroundings, so I guess you could say I have always had sympathy for the abused, the sad and those in pain. Many of our creatures were understandably nervous and I would do whatever I could to make them feel safe, secure and at home.

I was already 'talking' to animals from a young age and not questioning it, because why would I? Surely everyone can hear what their cat is saying to them? And hearing that the tortoise has a sore leg is normal, no? It wasn't until I got older that I realised this wasn't necessarily the case and I started to consciously listen.

Children definitely question less than adults, don't they? When we are young we see fairies, chat to trees, and completely accept the existence of different worlds that we consider to be fantasy when we are adults. It's a shame that we lose this when we get to an age where we're supposed to be grown-up and 'normal'. Who wants to be normal, anyway?

My horse career started young, as it does for so many of us. How can you not fall in love with such a strong, powerful, noble

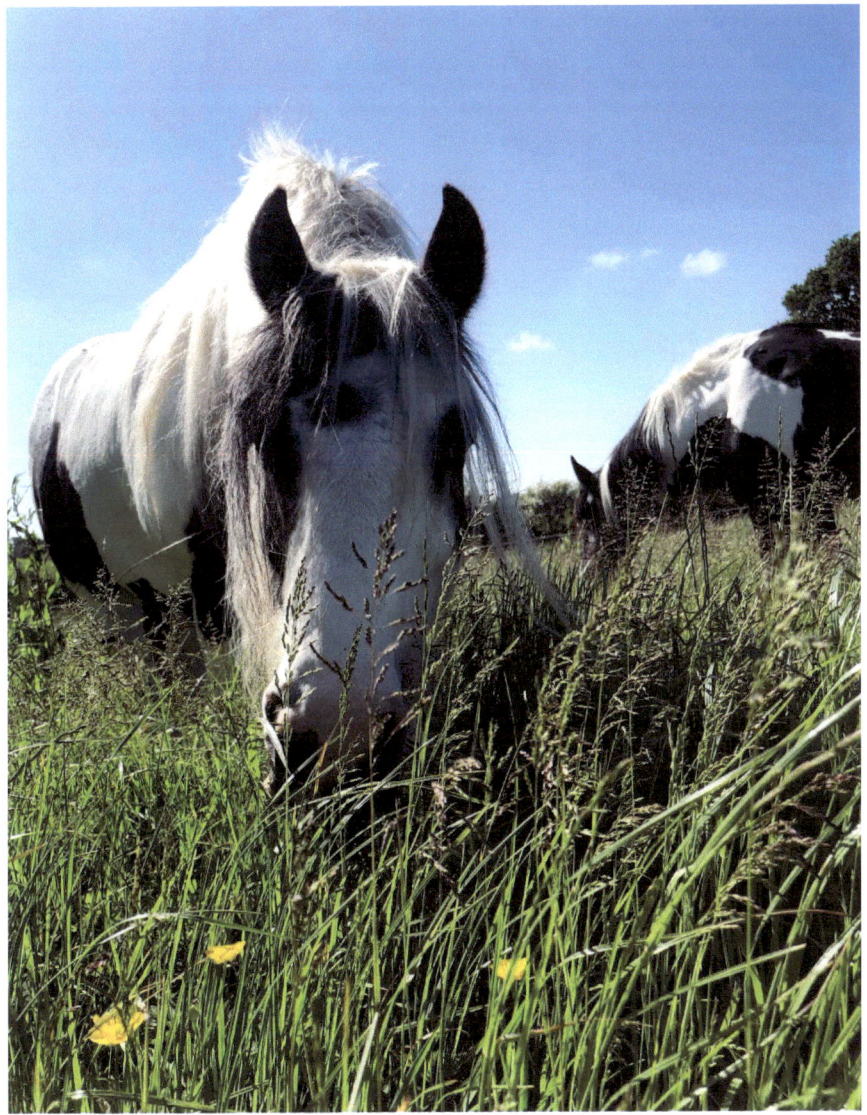

A 'heard' horse is a happy horse. (Anna Curtis)

creature? Yes, even Shetlands are strong, powerful and noble in their minds, even though they only reach halfway up the stable door!

I started riding enormous horses from a very young age, at a military base in Poole, Dorset. These horses were huge, being used for the military – and I was never an enormous person! Riding these big, strong horses has prepared me for facing some huge challenges in my life. My mum used to come home from a hack to find me wandering around the school, mounted on a 'mountain', in tears because I was being shouted at by military trainers who were used to big, burly men instead of a tiny seven-year-old girl. Although it was hard work, they taught me a lot about horses and I had a fantastic and thorough introduction to riding, for which I will always be grateful.

There were some amazing characters at the yard and I would have happily carried on riding them forever, however, because of my age, I wasn't allowed to hack out and was restricted to just schooling, but I had caught the horse bug and I couldn't imagine a life without horses and riding. This leads us neatly on to Ranger in the following chapter.

When I was around thirteen, I came across a series of books by Anne McCaffrey called *Dragonriders of Perne*. If you haven't read these fantastic stories, they're about humans who ride dragons and communicate with them telepathically. Anne McCaffrey was a horsey person and there have been comparisons drawn between the dragons and the equine species, which is not too surprising when you look at it. Communicating with horses is just about the only way to truly know them, experience them and connect with them – and it makes the rest of the working relationship, including the riding, so much more rewarding.

I'm not sure whether reading these books encouraged me to be more open to communicating with creatures in a language other than the spoken word, or if the books came to me because they were a clue to the direction that my life was going to take, but there is no doubt that they had a huge impact on me.

Having a good job that pays well is fine, but if it doesn't stir your soul and make you feel happy at least 50 per cent of the time, then it's not really worth it. Yes, I know we all have bills to pay and working at your dream job may not be practical or possible – but if a chance comes your way, you should grab it with both hands and not let go!

I had what most people would consider a good job; I was working in a bank, which paid well and kept me busy for the week. However, working in a bank is never going to be one of those things that stirs your soul though, is it? I enjoyed my non-work life considerably more, I had got into Tarot card readings and, through a chance encounter with a neighbour, I was training to be a reiki master.

Having done several readings for friends and family, my reputation as a 'psychic seer' was becoming established. I used to meet up with friends at their yards and would pass on what the horses were telling me. These friends mentioned me to other people and word of mouth was spreading. I soon had to hand in my notice at the bank, because I simply didn't have time to fit in the day job around the growing equine communicator work I was doing. Needless to say, life got better from then on! There is a lot to be said for a job that you love, which gives you fulfilment and satisfaction every single day. I genuinely love talking to your horses.

So, let's talk a little about the communicating itself. There is no special preparation, no gimmicks or rituals that I undertake to hear what the horse is saying – I can just hear them. Sometimes I still travel to meet the horses, but I find a photograph of the eye is just as effective. I'm sorry if you are reading this book wanting to be told, step by step, how I communicate with horses, and you are imagining a big reveal of the secret techniques and tricks I use, but I honestly cannot explain how I do it. I think a lot of it is to do with being open-minded, listening to that tiny inner voice and trusting your instincts – something we don't tend to do very much these days.

If you think about it, the majority of horse communication between herd members is silent. They use body language, facial expressions, and almost certainly their thoughts and feelings can be 'heard' by other members of the herd. This is why most of them are not surprised to be communicated with in the same way as they do with each other, although they often feel relief at finally being heard.

We know about horses' body language, right? We can watch how the herd interacts; we can tell if our horse is grumpy; we know when they are pleased to see us. Being open to this form of communication and allowing our horses the space and freedom to express themselves is a big part of what I do. I can fully imagine that you are also in tune with the moods of your horses; you know when there are days that they feel a little moody, or those days when they are filled with the joys of spring. Horses have different moods and feelings, just like we do.

I find often that a horse is very keen to talk to me. They are talking to us all the time; we just struggle to believe that there is any way of communicating beyond the spoken word. The truth is anyone can do this, you just have to remember what it was like that time you thought your horse was a little 'off', to then discover that they were coming down with something or hiding a cheeky hoof abscess. This is your – and their – inner voice trying to talk to you.

Can you do it? Yes, of course you can. I'll tell you a little more in subsequent chapters about the ways that you can make yourself more open to communicating with your horse, and what you can do to encourage open communication between the two of you. Remember there is absolutely nothing wrong with realising that you need outside help, whether that be from a vet, a bodyworker or an equine communicator – doing the best for the horses is what we all want, ultimately.

As horsey people, we know our horses inside out. Often, we have a stronger bond with them than we do with most people; they are our relaxation partners, joy bringers, therapists, challengers, teachers. Being open enough to know how they are feeling is not a big step on from this. I have always noticed, with every single client I've had, that people are actually *very* open to hearing what their horse is trying to say; there is usually a huge sense of relief from the owner as well as the horse that there is some sort of issue that can be worked on – something that can be fixed, as it were.

A horse who is in pain and is being asked, or forced, to continue to work through their pain, will react in the only way they can to express their discomfort – they will refuse to do what is being asked, or they will explode in a raging ball of bucking, kicking, rearing and biting. Being able to pinpoint what the problem is and help the horse and the owner work through it is just about the most satisfying part of my job.

Imagine being asked to do something that hurts you, while being surrounded by people who do not speak your language. You would probably first become upset, by the pain and the lack of understanding, then you might become angry. You are telling these people, in the best way you possibly can, that you are unhappy – yet they are not listening and are still forcing you to do whatever it is that is causing you pain. If they could sort out that niggling ache, or at least try to help you through what is scaring you so much, instead of blindly ignoring you, you would be much happier. But because they don't listen, or they don't seem to care, and they just keep telling you that you are bad, you decide the only way to make them stop hurting you is to hurt them back. You don't want to do this, it's not in your nature, but there really isn't any other option.

If I can get through to a horse that is considered difficult or dangerous, 100 per cent of the time there is a reason for their behaviour – whether it be past traumas, physical body issues, or even something as simple as disliking their nicknames! Horses are sentient beings, too, and if you don't like being called Fatty or Big Ears, why do you think a horse would feel any different?

Speaking of names, here's a tiny bugbear for you – it really rubs me up the wrong way when people refer to their horses as 'it'.

They are not inanimate objects; they are living, breathing, sentient beings. I always say that if you want an 'it' to take you around the place, get yourself a bike. 'It' in an affectionate way is one thing; 'it' in the way that completely removes and disregards a horse's sentience by a derogatory name is another.

Thankfully, we are seeing a slow change in the attitudes of the majority of the equine world; people are genuinely trying to understand their horses and do the very best for them that they possibly can. We have come a long way from the days of breaking horses, quite literally, and flogging them till they have no spirit left to fight back in any way.

I know that you care about your horses, you wouldn't be reading this book if you didn't want to understand them better and do your best for them. By paying attention to their needs, making sure that they are as happy and comfortable as possible – and by opening your mind to see beyond the basics that we all do on a daily basis, and realising that your horses are communicating with you all the time – you, too, can make your journey smoother and your horses happier.

3

RANGER

Everyone has a catalyst in their lives that points them on the path to doing what they are meant to be doing, right? In my case, unsurprisingly, it was a horse. He was my heart horse, my soulmate, the love of my life. He taught me so much and looking back I can see that he was my doorway into doing

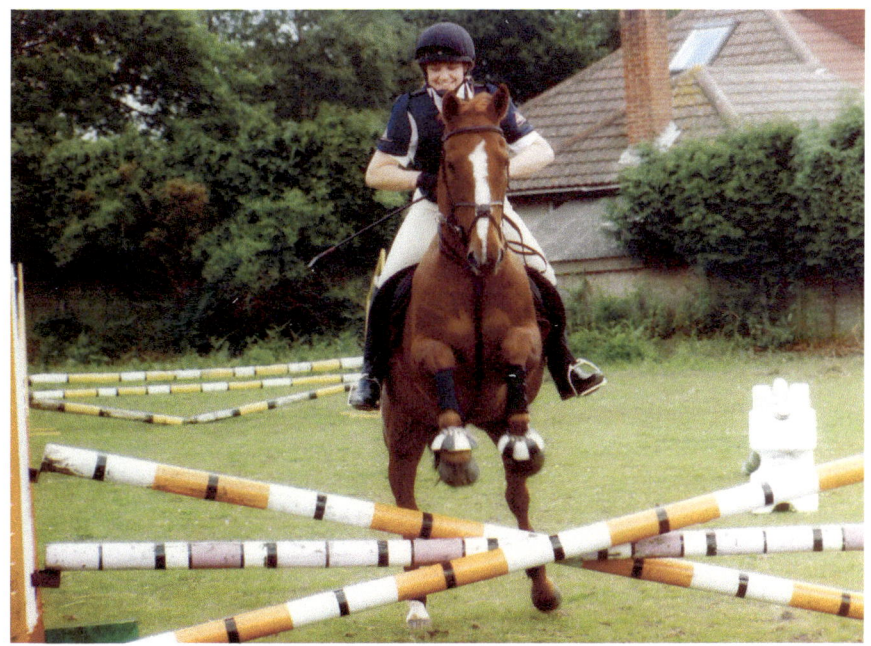

Ranger loved his work! (George 'Dusty' Miller, BEM, MSM)

what I do now. I would not be a full-time equine communicator had it not been for Ranger and I wouldn't have written this book. This is why he needs his own chapter, to immortalise him forever. I'll always be grateful for the times we spent together, and the things that have happened in my life as a consequence of knowing and loving him.

Ranger arrived in my life about the same time as the Anne McCaffrey books did when I was around thirteen. By then I was learning at a little riding school near Corfe Mullen, in Dorset, after having been first taught at the military school. As I was not allowed to take the military horses out due to my age, I had to find somewhere else to go hacking, so off I went to the riding school. In a field next to that school was a young horse called Ranger.

Ranger was a wild, unbroken, chestnut thoroughbred who was between eighteen months and two years old at the time. It was love at first sight. He wasn't enormous, but he had a heart the size of the universe. I knew that he was the one for me: his wild heart matched his personality!

My parents had always been very supportive of me, and when I started to ask for my own horse it was agreed that I could indeed have one, but I would be entirely responsible for buying said horse and doing absolutely everything to look after them. Well, we all know which horse I wanted! An unhandled thoroughbred, when I was barely out of childhood myself was possibly not the most logical choice. But he was my dream and I had to have him. We're all horse people; we have all experienced this type of madness, haven't we?

So, I lied about my age to secure a job working in McDonald's, and I scrimped and saved every penny I had. I worked weekends as a waitress and all the times outside school to save up the money to buy Ranger. I paid him off a little bit at a time. He was my sole focus; I just knew I had to have him with me. After months of saving and with the help of a small inheritance from my grandma, he was mine and I could finally bring him home. But the hard work didn't stop there.

The first time I put my own headcollar on him and got him into the field, I was then unable to catch him for the next three months. This horse made me work for it! I had to think up creative new ways to catch him just about every day. One of the main things he taught me was patience. Patience, as we all know, is something you have to have in bucketfuls when you are working with horses, especially youngsters – and it's not something I naturally possess! But we work the hardest and try our most for the things that we want above everything else, and Ranger was all I wanted.

I would be out of the house and up at the yard by 5 a.m. to muck out and care for Ranger, and in the later years when he was started under saddle I would also ride him. I was always back home by 7 a.m., to be ready for school and work. I was not too demanding of my parents; those early morning rides were after I could ride my moped or drive my car. Ranger kept me on the straight and narrow as I got older – yes, I would still have nights out with my friends, but the first thing I would do in the morning was sort out my horse – only then would I come home and nurse my hangover! I don't think I would have gone completely off the rails without Ranger – it's not entirely in my nature – but I do know I may have skated a little too close to the edge without my beloved four-legged anchor.

Ranger was a force of nature. He always knew exactly what he wanted and he would make me work for every little victory, but my God, it was so rewarding. Once I had figured out that I had to be creative with catching him, he would let me catch him easily 99 per cent of the time, but no one else was allowed to do so.

It was clear from the start that 'traditional' methods wouldn't work with this horse. He was too intelligent and too stubborn. I had to find my way into his brain somehow. I bought books on horse psychology and devoured them from cover to cover. I found new ways to connect with him, and we found our way together. Once we'd established our groove, I set about starting him – if I had known then what I know now, I would have left him to mature for longer – but we started our riding career together when Ranger was rising four. I worked him entirely by myself, using my experience with horses and my instincts.

Interestingly, despite the fact that he was such a difficult horse later in life, Ranger was very easy to break. We took it pretty slowly, introducing him to new things then leaving him in the field to process them for a while, then some more new information, then back to resting. He just took everything in his stride, from getting used to traffic to putting up with me leaning over his back, getting him used to tack and the feel of having someone on board.

I remember finally getting on his back and asking him to walk forward, and he never batted an eyelid! He was the most forgiving and understanding horse. My parents used to walk out with me on our first rides, just to keep an eye and make sure everything was safe – even in the 1980s there were idiots on the road.

We took it very gradually, of course. I still had to fit in school, work and a social life, after all, and Ranger would not be rushed. By the time he was fully trained up, he could have quietly ridden down the middle of the M27 during rush hour, but he still had his quirks. He would plant his feet and refuse to budge an inch if he spotted something in the distance he didn't like. He would turn inside out at the sight of a crisp packet flapping six miles away. In familiar surroundings I could do absolutely anything with him, but if I took him too far from home he would completely lose his marbles.

He developed a reputation in our local area, people called him 'dangerous' and more than once I was told that he should be shot. I knew better though. This horse and I communicated with each other right from the start – I even taught him to tap his hoof to say 'please!' I was still learning about my own gifts, and it seemed like a good cross-over to get him to 'say' something that people could instantly understand.

Ranger was already communicating with me, although I wasn't as open to it then as I am now. As an example, I was out for the day with my then boyfriend, when I stopped in the middle of the road and blurted out, 'I've got to get to the field, something's horribly wrong!'

My boyfriend looked at me as if I was mad, and tried to talk me out of it, but I was adamant that my horse needed me. When we got there, Ranger was standing quietly in the field, with barbed wire wrapped tightly around three of his legs, and with a gaping abdominal wound. He let me help him and with the essential vet treatment he was soon on the road to recovery. This experience made me realise even more the close bond we had, and I was so grateful that I had been able to hear his calls for help.

He would express his displeasure at being asked to do something that he didn't want to by rearing; a friend once counted twelve perfectly vertical back foot stands when we were out on a hack together! Yes, he did go over backwards sometimes. Unbelievably, he never put me in hospital. He always knew exactly where I was at any given time and even when we were both scraping ourselves up off the floor, he would look back at me as if to check that his calculations were right.

The years went by like this and Ranger was always my constant – friends, jobs and men would come and go – my horse was always there for me. I had a couple of long-term relationships and even went as far as getting engaged and buying a flat, then my fiancé said to me one day, 'If you sell that horse, we'll be able to afford a really nice three-piece suite!'

I was gobsmacked! I didn't make a decision right there and then, but the following morning I packed my things, broke off the engagement and let him buy me out of the flat. Luckily, I hadn't yet completely moved in, but I had to cancel all the wedding arrangements. Of course, Ranger was there waiting for me. He got me through everything.

When I was about fifteen, I remember coming down the stairs in floods of tears. I told my mum that I'd had a dream where Ranger had broken his leg and had to be destroyed. It felt so real; I could hardly believe that he was still with me, out in the field. Then, on 18 May 2000, I realised that this had been a prophetic dream. When Ranger died and it was the end of our physical journey together, it almost broke me.

The night before he died, he didn't want to come in. I didn't think much of it; this was a recurring theme throughout his life – he'd always been difficult to catch. It was a beautiful May evening, he was in the field with his big chestnut friend and he was just having too much fun. I decided to leave him to it; what could possibly go wrong? As I drove away from the field, I looked in the rear-view mirror and saw him doing one of his signature vertical rears – he was so happy and free, and living his best life.

That night I was sitting at home, ten minutes away from the field, and I had a feeling that I should go and get him in at about midnight. I decided not to because there was absolutely no indication that anything was wrong – and if I got him in, I'd have to also bring in his field mate who wasn't mine and, as it was a shared yard, I didn't want to step on any toes. The next day I got to the field at about 5.30 a.m., to find Ranger standing at the gate. Then he moved slightly, and I could suddenly see that nearly the whole of his off-side fore below the knee was completely severed. There was no vet who could have done anything at all to save him with that horrific injury.

I fell to the ground in shock and horror, crying and screaming, before calling everyone including the vet – who came and told me what I already knew. I had him put down by injection and I remember sending everyone away, even my mum – this moment was between me and my horse. It had always been just us and our extraordinary bond, and I wanted him to go on his way with me right by his side, without the complications and emotions of other people. The last thing I could do for him was to be with him when he died. His passing was so peaceful, despite the traumatic experiences leading up to it, which is something I'm grateful for.

I was twenty-eight and Ranger was seventeen when he died and the bottom fell out of my entire world. Nothing was ever the same again. He was the most amazing, perfectly bonded, special horse. Not all of us are fortunate enough to have this bond, but if you have ever found your own heart horse then you will know exactly what I mean. I'd gone through so much in my life to that point – from divorce to illnesses to friendship issues and family problems – and sailed through them, because I had my Ranger by my side. I still cry about him, even twenty-three years on. I feel him around me constantly. I can communicate with many different people and horses, but there is one thing I will never be able to communicate and that is my unending love for Ranger and how much I miss him, every single day.

This book is for Ranger, and for every other horse that is considered to be dangerous or difficult; the ones that are en route to the last chance saloon; the ones that could be destroyed needlessly, but who can be saved with love, compassion and understanding.

4

BODYWORKERS

In the same way that it takes a village to raise a child, it takes a village to ensure that a horse is as happy as he or she can be. You might think that now you have the horse, you can just get on and enjoy it, and there will never be a single problem as long as you both live, right?

Um, no, actually. It's a very lucky horse owner who has not had to shell out thousands for the vet, or who doesn't feel like they're literally feeding fifty-pound notes to their horses.

So, you have a horse – this means that you also have to have an army of other people to help your horse be their best. You will have a farrier, a vet, a dentist and a saddle fitter. Maybe a chiropractor, a Bowen therapist, or perhaps an osteopath – and the list goes on.

All these people, highly qualified and experienced in their own different ways, do their best to make sure your horse is as healthy and happy as they can be physically, while you look after the mental side of things and get on with the fun aspects, like the bonding, playtime, grooming, riding – generally loving your horse and doing what you and they like to do best.

I'm not saying that bodywork is absolutely essential for every single horse – like some people, there will be horses who go

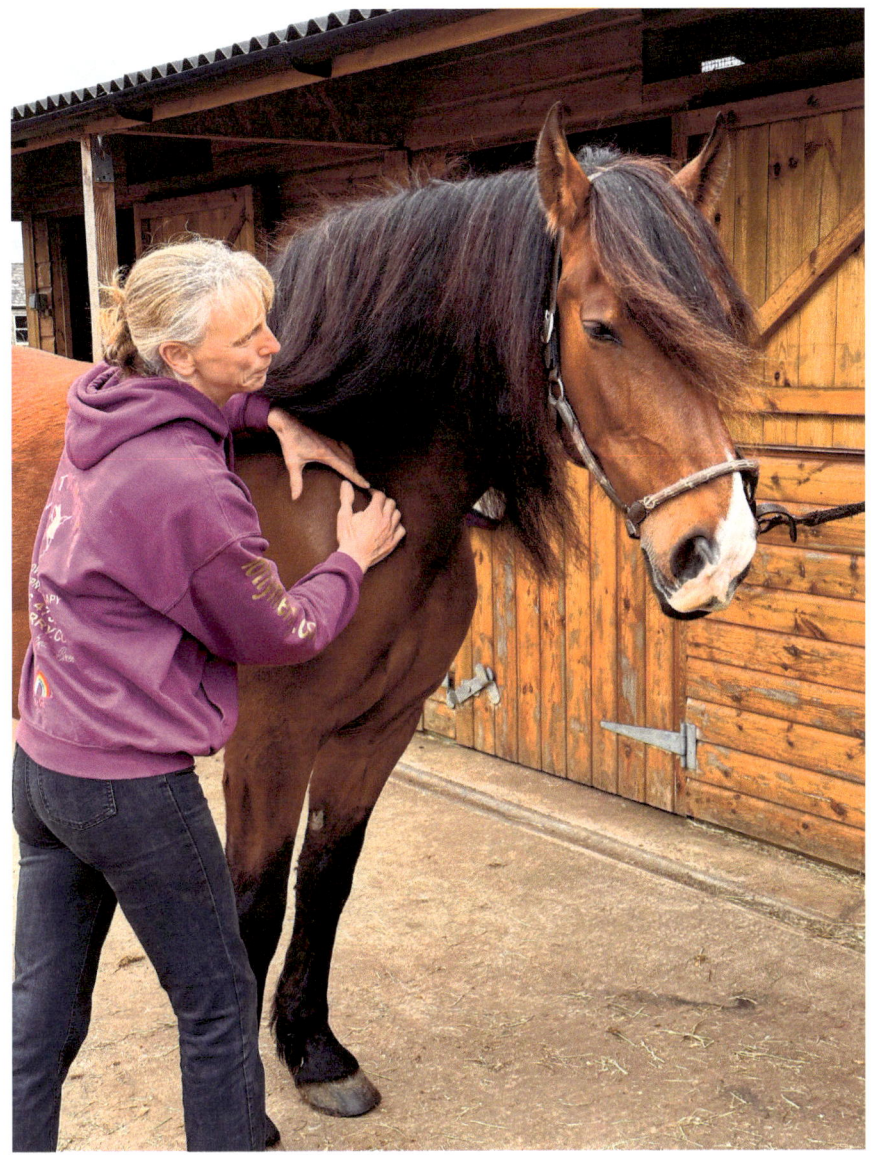

An equine therapist can help with so many physical issues. (Lotty Merry)

through life without a single injury, ache or pain. However, we know that this is pretty unlikely, for horses and humans – and if you're over thirty you'll already be starting to know what I mean! Even if your horse appears to be in perfect physical health, there is nothing wrong – and in fact everything right – with giving them a good once-over from a trained professional every once in a while.

Retired horses living in fields can slip and pick up injuries; horses in intensive work regimes can get stiff and achy. We have all sorts of sports physios and masseurs for people, and horses should be no different – there are a lot of things you can do to help your horse feel more comfortable. Because they cannot express with words that their left stifle is locking up, or that they have deep muscle trauma from that extra-large cross-country jump, we may not know there is a problem until they tell us with explosive behaviour or a refusal to work.

I work closely with several bodyworkers – people who are attuned to the physical side of the horse and can help with problems of the muscles, bones, digestive system, hooves, and just about everything else. I find that this is an essential part of what I do – I can find out what the problem is, but I am not a qualified osteopath or equine dental technician, and I have no desire to be up to my elbows in a horse's mouth, filing down sharp teeth!

I often identify a problem in the physical body of the horse, meaning that I can then recommend treatment by a professional who is qualified and experienced to deal with the problem. My favourite recommendation is Bowen therapy (more on this later) as it works with both the physical and the emotional sides of the horse, and it can fix myriad problems that often leave vets scratching their heads.

I am *very* vocal about working in conjunction with bodyworkers, vets, saddle fitters, dentists, and the army of people that help horses be as happy and as comfortable as they can be. I feel that what I do can be used as another diagnostic tool, particularly when – as happens in so many cases – the routine scans, tests and checks don't show up the problem. We are all in this together for our horses; we should not be working in competition with each other. All of us are striving for the best outcome for horses and owners alike.

Without this holistic approach to treating a horse's problems, many owners would still be at the same impasse they were when they first called on me. I am incredibly grateful to the bodyworkers I work with; many of them started out being extremely sceptical (who wouldn't be surprised to hear that a horse, who looks perfectly fine on the outside, has a problem with his sacroiliac joint that cannot be found by any vet?), but are now firmly on the side of communication between me and the horse.

I am indebted to those who look after the horse's physical well-being, once the horse has told me where in his body the problem is situated. Someone who is highly trained and qualified to deal with physical problems that a horse can identify to me is essential to what I do – making horses feel better. We are all cogs in a wheel and I am honoured to be a part of this. As we have continued to work together, other professionals have become more understanding and accepting of what I do. Like me, they can't explain it. Like me, they know it works.

My favourite practitioner is Marion Watts, who fits into both the Bowen therapist and the massively sceptical boxes. Marion will openly admit that she has been trying to prove me wrong in what I do for all the years we have worked together; happily, for us both, she has not yet managed to do this and we continue to work together to fix the problems of the horses that we deal with.

There are a great many benefits to all the different types of bodywork, depending on the horse and their particular needs. Whatever therapist you can find who can make a difference to your horse's physical and mental well-being is fantastic – just make sure that you always check for qualifications, credentials and reviews.

No horse wakes up in the morning and thinks to themselves, 'I wonder what I can do today that will cement my reputation as a total nuisance?' There is always a reason for their bad behaviour and a lot of the time it is to do with being in pain. Working with equine therapists can enable us to get to the root of the problem and help the horses – and the owners – immeasurably.

This is where I and communication with the horse can really help, because the horse can relay the issue and essentially be heard. Working together to help the horse, can speed up the process and improve the outcome for everyone. On a daily basis most horses are well-balanced individuals who get five-star care and want for nothing, but some, despite this, will have a moment in the lorry, trailer, stable, field or competition. They may slip, slide, fall, get cast, get kicked or have an accident – sometimes we don't even know it's happened, and are left guessing how three broken fence posts and a 15-metre skid occurred in the night.

Rescue horses often have a lifetime of trauma behind them, which can lead to less-favourable behaviour such as aggression (based on fear) and practitioners can risk reactions of biting, kicking and squashing. This work can actually be dangerous for a bodyworker and I find that communicating with the horse while treatment is taking place is very beneficial. Remember that horses are flight animals and by treating the horse we may inadvertently make it feel like it is losing control. I always have to be aware that the owner has requested treatment, not the horse, and work sensitively with everyone in order to get the best results.

Often when trauma occurs, the brain can almost zone out to the pain signals it gets, using other areas to compensate and create new movement patterns. These new patterns can often result in compromised ability, resulting in pain, discomfort, and a lack of performance. This new pattern and atrophy can take a while to show, and during this time, potentially, the body is using more and more muscle in areas not designed to withstand that type of work, creating asymmetry, which, in turn, will possibly affect saddle fit, foot balance and rider stability. This shows you how very important it is to treat symptoms of pain or discomfort in your horse – it will actually help you in the long run, too.

I am often the last resort for people who are having problems with their horses. They have tried the vet route, they've gone to every bodyworker they can find, they've had expensive scans and tests done, which show that there is nothing wrong. I can rock up in a yard, tell an owner that their horse is being crucified by the fit of their saddle, or that they've had neck pain for months, or their back is out of alignment – and the owner will *still* say, 'Oh, well I've got this competition booked for Sunday, can I still do that?' The answer is *no*! If you can hear, albeit through someone else, that your horse is in severe pain (and has usually still been trying their heart out to please you despite the agony), then you *do* something about it!

Do your horse a favour – if a problem has been identified, do everything you can to try and fix it – even if this involves using a type of bodywork that you feel sceptical about, or have never used before. Your horse, your riding career, and your relationship with your horse will all benefit massively.

It's okay to use a variety of different treatments for your horse; if you favour both McTimoney and Bowen, the two can be used together and you won't find that they counteract each other. Just ensure that you give your horse plenty of time between each treatment to allow the adjustments from one to settle before you start with another.

Before I go any further, I must stress a vital point and that is if your horse has a problem, then you must *always* get it diagnosed by a vet *first*. You can follow whatever type of treatment you like afterwards – massage, Bowen, physiotherapy or McTimoney – but make sure you have investigated all possibilities with your vet before you decide on a course of treatment.

Physiotherapy

In the same way that we humans benefit from having someone who is highly qualified to know which part of the body is feeling pain, and what to do about it, horses are great candidates for physiotherapy. Horse physiotherapy actually derived from human physiotherapy; practitioners are experts in knowing which part of the body is causing problems, and the types of movements to prescribe to help fix them.

All physiotherapists qualify on a course that teaches them about human physiology and anatomy; equine physiotherapists go on to specifically study the physiology and anatomy of horses. These people really know bodies. They can tell you what to do if a load-bearing joint is inflamed and they can give you the best plan to rehabilitate your horse back into work after an injury.

Physiotherapy can help with soft-tissue injuries, skeletal problems, nerve injuries, wounds, scar tissue, and general joint stiffness. It is one of the more traditional treatments that I would recommend to clients and is more suitable for those horses who don't mind being handled and physically manipulated by strangers. Those who have a little more 'stranger danger', or who have been known to be aggressive and dislike touch would definitely be better with one of the more hands-off treatments.

Physiotherapists can also give you specific exercises to do with your horse, to help improve the problem and stop it recurring. As I have said before, if someone gives you a recommendation of things to do to improve your horse, do it. I know that gentle walking and stretching exercises are not necessarily what you want to be doing with your eventer, but you should definitely give them a go.

Massage
Who doesn't love a good massage? There's nothing like having those sore muscles stretched and manipulated and gently eased back into position. Massage helps to soothe, soften and relax the muscle tissues, and it can also help to realign them if they have slipped out of position or are becoming inflamed.

Massage is a great technique to either warm up or cool down your horse, before or after exercise. It's also a great thing for helping establish a connection between you and your horse, but you do need to be careful with it! Giving your horse's back a quick rub is all very well, but it's best to get a professional involved if you think your horse has some really tight muscles and ligaments that need releasing.

It can aid those horses who have problems with flexibility; this is one of the key things that helps them move comfortably and easily and can reduce pain. You may even find that your horse's suppleness improves after a few sessions of professional massage. Because massage is targeted towards the muscles, it is a great therapy for horses who are involved in heavy work and need the muscles to recover between sessions.

Massage can also pinpoint areas where the rider is unbalanced; if you are regularly riding your horse and your posture is off, the chances are they will adapt themselves to hold you straight. If your horse is consistently unbalanced on one side, your masseur might be able to give you some tips on your riding position which will help you both.

Regular massage can also help enormously with your horse's mental well-being. We all know about the benefits of relaxing. Well, it's exactly the same for your horse. When they are relaxed, there is far less adrenaline running through the body, which will lead to them being less anxious and reactive in daily life.

Generally, the end of a massage will feature a sweeping motion along all the areas that have been focused on – this is extremely beneficial as it aids with the flow of the lymphatic fluid towards the lymph nodes, which helps to remove stored-up toxins in the body.

Bowen
This is a rather magical technique, which is used to treat a variety of problems with the joints and muscles, and it can help with

injuries sustained on the job as well – it is ideal for horses that do a lot of competing, or hard work such as racing or cross-country. Of course, it can also be used on our field ornaments that have somehow injured themselves by standing around in the field, too!

Bowen therapy is definitely my 'drug of choice' to treat just about anything in a horse, as it is a holistic approach – that is, it takes into account the whole body, and fixes the underlying cause of the problems, rather than just putting a plaster over them. It is a brilliantly subtle way of getting communication between the horse's body and its brain, the moves are gentle, and it sometimes seems like nothing is happening at all – but Bowen therapy is a series of specific moves, connecting the external messaging system through the nerve endings of the skin and muscles, all the way to the central control centre, the brain.

Bowen therapy uses techniques of gently manipulating the soft tissues and connective tissues around the muscles in a very specific way. I am not one of these wonderful people, but I do have a few trusted practitioners that I will recommend to clients if I pick up that the horse has a muscular or joint problem. Bowen is very gentle, so it is ideal for horses who are particularly sensitive to touch or manipulation.

As well as improving pain and mobility, Bowen can help improve our horses' mental states, as it can also be used for treating stress and improving the general well-being of a horse. Stress is a huge factor in these prey animals' behavioural issues, so having someone able to help with their mental state is invaluable. Bowen can even assist with riding confidence, competing, jumping, open spaces, or any other issues – physical or mental – that the horse may present with, such as the phobia of spiders in the tack room, disliking mirrors in the school, etc.

Bowen can help the body to realign itself, to regain the connection within and re-establish the correct message pathways. While Bowen never purports to 'fix' things, it can support the body along the way and encourage it to make the adjustments needed, as part of a rehabilitation or work plan including the vet, trainer, farrier and saddle fitter.

The subtlety of Bowen is the key, with a gentle touch the body is more likely to absorb the information given, without feeling the need to tense or become defensive. This is really important with horses who have had trauma. Their systems are already on alert, their flight mechanisms are maxed out and the cells are under stress, so creating a strong input to this already loaded system would potentially result in the horse contracting its muscles and recoiling rather than releasing and absorbing. Pain creates contraction.

The reactions to a successful Bowen treatment are often very noticeable – favourites are really deep, heartfelt sighs; yawning (once they start you'll often get fifteen to twenty and more); eyes closing, and even dozing off. Horses and people often feel tired during and after treatment as the internal systems are now firing, leaving a rather vacant external look. It's nothing to worry about! Other reactions include lymph stripes, snoring, stretches (and they can do some radical yoga poses mid-treatment), face pulling, swaying, and even lying down.

Emmett

The Emmett technique has been practised on horses in the UK since 2011, and it is a highly effective form of treatment for all sorts of things – from rehabilitation, behavioural issues and injuries, to general health and well-being.

Emmett works by applying pressure to specific 'Emmett points' on the body, which helps to release muscle tension and improve movement. It does all this in an incredibly gentle, non-invasive way, which is almost always received favourably by the horse.

Interestingly, the Emmett points are not the same as acupressure or acupuncture points – they are unique to the Emmett technique – and the movements used to trigger these points are incredibly light and gentle. This technique works well, especially on those horses who are averse to touch or to more uncomfortable manipulations.

An Emmett practitioner knows where the points are on the body that can reset the horse's muscle tension; the touches on the Emmett points relay messages to the brain which can help the muscles to settle themselves back into a more favourable position.

Owners report that their horses can react almost instantly to this technique, showing release by yawning and stretching. They generally benefit from a session and even things like behavioural issues can be improved.

McTimoney

This is a branch of chiropractic treatment – but it is not the 'crack, crunch!' type of chiropractic therapy that involves manipulating limbs and making things click back into place. Like the others listed in this section, it can be practised on people as well as animals, and horses tend to respond exceptionally well to this type of treatment.

Despite the title, McTimoney chiropractic is not just about dealing with backs and spines. It works on a gentle release of the spinal cord, where all the nerves run down in pairs off each vertebral joint. Where there is muscle tightness or a restriction that causes the vertebrae to slip out of alignment, the joint space is reduced and the tiny exit hole for the nerves gets even smaller, causing nerve pain in that area, which can then spread to other parts of the body – the internal organs as well as the muscles.

McTimoney is a whole-body technique that helps to realign the musculoskeletal system, using a series of very specific movements. Watching a treatment you would be forgiven for thinking that nothing was really happening, the movements are so subtle, but just wait until you see the difference in your horse afterwards! They often 'release' during a treatment – yawning and relaxing – and some even nod off. If you get the right practitioner, McTimoney is nothing short of miraculous.

Removing pain is just about the most effective way of getting past behavioural and ridden issues, so this is something I often recommend to clients – especially if the problem is related to the skeleton rather than the muscles – although McTimoney is effective in this, too.

If the internal structure of the body – the scaffolding that holds it all together – is out of whack then no amount of stretching, massage or corrective riding will help to fix the problem. Delving deeper into the problem and using McTimoney's gentle adjustments will help enormously.

Reiki

This is a Japanese form of healing that uses the flow of energy based on chakras. Practitioners can use a hands-on method to guide healing energy through the body, which reduces stress and encourages good health, or reiki can be performed from a distance. Reiki is used for treating physical issues, but it can also treat those in the non-physical body, too, such as stress and emotional problems. It is a holistic approach that aims to treat the whole being, not just a part of the body.

Reiki is fabulous for horses and people alike. It can be especially effective for horses that are too wild or who don't like being touched, or those whose pain is too great for them to allow anyone near enough to treat them, because the treatment can be done from a distance. Reiki can even travel across the world; I remember one session working on a horse in New South Wales, Australia, while sitting in my living room in Wimborne, Dorset!

I first got into reiki in 2011, inspired by my neighbour, Debbie, who offered to attune me. I did my reiki 1, 2 and 3 with Debbie and was taught on people, but I did my reiki attunement with a wonderful farrier and I always had horses in my mind. I wasn't trained for animals, but the practice of reiki is the same for animals and people as the chakras are in the same places, and the principle is the same.

There are many fantastic bodyworkers out there, and you can work your way through them and find out which type is best for you and for your horse. It's always good to ask around and take recommendations from your friends or your vet – a good review goes a long way, and you will find those with the most favourable reviews are generally the best. Or, if you want to learn, you can go on any number of courses and become a fully qualified bodyworker yourself. There are courses available for each and every one of these therapies, and although it might be a costly start-up, it can lead to great things in the future. Maybe you, like me, will find your true calling in an alternative therapy.

5

GUT FEELINGS

They say, 'you are what you eat' and this is true of both horses and people. If you go about your life living on nothing but junk food, cake, black coffee and wine, your body will eventually start to protest. Horses are more complicated than us in terms of their digestion and what they can and cannot eat, but the same thing applies – diet is *massively* important for good health.

It is becoming increasingly prevalent in many studies that good gut health is linked to the brain, the nervous system, attitudes and behaviour. Remember the fact that some children go absolutely wild when they ingest a certain type of E number? What we put into our bodies really does affect our minds – and horses are no different.

In the wild, horses spend the majority of their days grazing. In fact, they can graze between fifteen and seventeen hours per day! Horses are non-ruminant animals – meaning they only have one stomach, unlike cows – but their digestive system really should be thought of as being in two parts: horses digest their food enzymatically in the foregut, then it ferments in the hindgut. This is a very basic explanation, but you can find any amount of additional information online or in books; I never claimed to be an equine nutritionist!

There are a number of recent studies showing the link between diet and the mind for horses and people; it is becoming more widely accepted that the gut is a huge part of the nervous system, and that the whole body is connected.

Horses are designed to consume small amounts of food, very regularly, but with our busy lifestyles and the way we keep our horses this is not always possible. The most natural diet you can feed your horse is grass, but this is a tricky subject. The grass that is available to them is not what they would be used to as wild creatures; we have fields full of fatty, sugary rye grass, rather than the 'pick' that horses would find in their natural habitat. In the wild, the grass would be sparser, much lower in sugars and containing a huge variety of different grasses and other plants.

Grazing itself can be quite difficult nowadays. Some liveries don't allow all-year-round turnout; you may not have a big enough field and you need to strip graze; or perhaps your horse is on a restricted diet for health reasons.

Many horses are kept at livery, meaning they are necessarily restricted from grazing as they naturally would, so we have to do our best to make sure that they are able to continue eating in a way that keeps them healthy. Sometimes this means unlimited access to hay, or strip grazing to get as much nutrition from what's available as possible, and even supplementing with hard feed can be another way to ensure our horses get all the right nutrition.

With this in mind, what is the best thing that you can feed your horse? Well, as natural as possible is the ideal, but many of us don't have the luxury to just let our horses out on to a hillside and allow them to make the most of it. So, grass and grazing are the best things, but we also have to watch out for obesity and laminitis. If you have to keep your horse on limited turnout then you will be familiar with hay feeding regularly (aka constantly!) and this is the best thing that you can do for your horse in these circumstances. Hay is dried grass; okay they wouldn't necessarily find it in the wild, but if it's what we have to feed them, then that's what we'll use.

Hay is incredibly good for horses; not only is it simply a dried version of what they would naturally eat in the wild, but it also provides energy and a great deal of fibre and roughage, something that is essential for a horse's digestion. In the same way as with grass, there are better and worse versions, so do try to ensure that your hay supplier doesn't use any pesticides or chemicals on the crop, and watch out for mouldy bales as these won't do your horse any good.

So, we have horses that are restricted to certain areas of grazing at particular times, and we try our hardest to keep them as naturally as we can, but this is difficult with our restrictions. If supplementing our horses with hard feed is something else we can do to help their gut – and therefore general – health, then we need to make sure this is also of the best quality for the best results. If your horse is regularly given hard feed, there are a few things that you really should bear in mind.

Now, for obvious reasons, I'm not going to name any names, but there is a type of horse food that seems to cause more hindgut issues and gastric ulcers than any other. I can *always* tell if a horse has been fed this particular brand, and clients are often surprised when I can name the contents of their feed room – this is because I can feel it in the horse. They are in pain, their digestion is not functioning as it should be, and they are generally far less healthy than horses who do not eat this type of food.

All I will say for now is, in my experience, when I pick up hindgut issues or other stomach discomfort, a whopping 95 per cent of the time it is related to the chaff that fills most of the bucket. Great care and attention should be given to the texture of the chaff you are feeding; a coarse chaff tends to irritate the hindgut or the stomach lining and can lead to ulcers. Feed a softer, finer chaff whenever you can.

Fortunately, horse food is improving. It has come a long way from the days when it was scrapings from a factory floor and loaded with molasses to make it even halfway edible. Nowadays, manufacturers are leaning towards the more natural, forage-based feeds and they are becoming much healthier for your horse. As we gain awareness, more feeds are available that are organic and non-GMO, but you still have to keep an eye on the ingredients list.

Balancers are another tricky subject. People use them to supplement horses to ensure that they get the right balance of vitamins and minerals that is often lacking in our grass but, unfortunately, many of them are not actually very beneficial at all. If you do want to use one, you should find the most natural version that you can, which doesn't contain GMO ingredients. Another thing to bear in mind is that balancers are often high in magnesium, which is something that very few horses are deficient in.

Obviously, what each horse needs to eat depends on their body type, their workload and their general health issues, so you will have to work out what food your horse needs based on their individual requirements. That being said, if you do feed your horses hard feed, there are a few things you can do to make it all-round healthier for them, and to help ensure they are getting all the right nutrients from their food that they would normally get from a 100 per cent grass diet. Along with decent chaff, feeding supplements is another thing that we can do to help keep our horses healthy. As standard, there are a few things that you should think about putting in their buckets.

Many of these things are not what horses would naturally forage for if they were still running wild across the plains, but then again, neither is hay or chaff! A little note on the supplements – do your homework and make sure that you are buying the best quality. Check *all* the ingredients. Some contain things that you wouldn't want to be feeding your horses; some are not as high quality as they could be, and some contain fillers that basically cancel out the benefit of the supplements. As always, I'm not going to name names, but just make sure you look into things thoroughly.

Garlic

As you may already know, garlic has myriad health benefits for both humans and animals. It is a blood purifier and a very good all-round immune booster, plus it can improve the appetite, reduce the blood pressure and is a natural source of methylsulfonylmethane (MSM) which can be used to treat joint problems and allergies. Horses fed with garlic supplements may also be less susceptible to flies, as they sweat out the smell of the garlic that flies don't like. It also has antimicrobial properties when applied to the skin, but this should be done with the *utmost caution*, as raw garlic can burn and blister the skin. You can buy any amount of garlic powder, which is the best way to get it into your horse – just start off slowly, if you have never fed it before. Begin with 1 teaspoon sprinkled over a feed for three days, then increase to 2 teaspoons for three days and so on, but make sure to not exceed 9 teaspoons per day, as too much garlic can cause health problems.

Turmeric

This is a wonder, which should be fed to each and every one of us and our horses! Its primary use is for anti-inflammatory properties, and it can be used to treat arthritis and laminitis fairly successfully. It can also help skin conditions, the respiratory system and even digestive issues and liver function. There are no real upper limits on how much turmeric you can feed to your horses, as there have been no adverse effects recorded, but it is sensible to stick to a dose of around 2g a day. Horses have been treated with up to 20g per day for short periods of time, again with no adverse effects recorded, but it is wise to stick to a smaller dose, especially if you have not fed it before and your horse is not used to the fairly strong flavour.

Seaweed

The humble seaweed is actually a powerhouse of goodness, for both you and your horse. It is an excellent source of iodine, making it a great choice for a feed supplement if your horse has thyroid issues. It is also a great source of prebiotics, which can help them digest soluble fibre better, and can even increase the absorption of other minerals and supplements you add to their feed. Seaweed can also improve your horse's coat and hooves, and also help their performance. It is recommended that you feed around 10g per 100kg of bodyweight, for best results – but again, you cannot really overdose on this.

Vitamins

Horses, especially those who are kept in without access to grass, may need supplementing with vitamins. Most of the vitamins necessary for horses' optimal health come from the grass and hay they forage daily, but if your hay is soaked or your grazing is limited then you may have to supplement. Vitamin A is especially important for a stabled horse, as they usually get the right amount of this from fresh grass, which is rich in it. You can find a good vitamin A supplement pretty easily. Vitamin C is very good for the immune system – it helps to build immunity against disease and can help reduce inflammation. B vitamins are important for good hoof health, but generally horses can synthesise B vitamins in their bodies. There are very rarely cases of horses suffering B12 deficiencies, as they tend to get enough from their forage.

Salt

This electrolyte is the most important mineral in your horse's diet. Horses' bodies are around 70 per cent fluid, including water and electrolytes, and this balance of fluids needs to be kept at an optimal level for things to run smoothly. If sodium levels in the body are too low, the brain will not register that it needs to drink, and your horse can go downhill very rapidly. This is because the brain knows that taking on more water will dilute the sodium levels, so it removes the thirst response. Salt also plays a crucial part in ensuring proper nerve function and the essential digestive tract, as well as urine, sweat and saliva. Using a salt-lick is one way to get salt into your horses, but they generally don't get enough of this vital mineral from salt-licks alone.

Water

I know this is not a supplement, but I had to include it because this is just about the single most important thing you can make sure your horse has access to. Like the rest of us, horses cannot survive for long without water. Horses will drink between 6 and 10 gallons of water every day, and up to 15 in hot weather. Working horses can go through as much as 18 gallons of water a day, so access to water is vitally important. They must always have free access to fresh, clean water. If your horse is kept in a field without a trough, or they need to be kept in for long periods, prepare to visit several times a day to make sure they have enough to drink. Without enough clean water, your horse's body will start to fall apart alarmingly quickly.

Water is something that you can also use to increase your horse's intakes of certain vitamins and minerals; adding a few buckets containing water mixed with turmeric, apple cider vinegar, bicarbonate of soda or rosehips, for example, can really give their health a boost.

More and more studies are coming to light that show a direct link between the gut microbiome and potential behavioural issues. Horses in test studies that were fed a diet much higher in starch have been shown to exhibit 'spooky' behaviour, and to seem as though they are 'on their toes'. This is not very surprising, when we consider that we really *are* what we eat, and that there is such an important connection between the central nervous system and the intestinal tract.

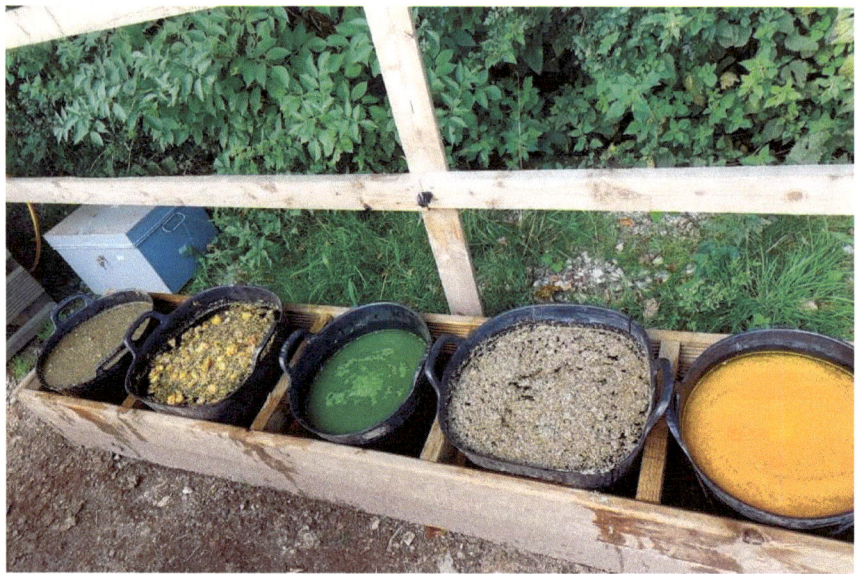

Horses love having tasty, healthy additions to their water. (The Cornish Ranch Track Livery)

Interestingly, a diet high in starch has been shown to reduce the fibre-fermenting bacteria in a horse's gut (that's Ruminococcaceae, in case you were wondering), and as horses' diets are primarily fibre, this can only cause them problems. Horses fed a higher starch diet are far more susceptible to colic and laminitis, as well as the behavioural issues that we have already mentioned.

Of course, horses in high-performance jobs are going to need a little extra in their diets, in the form of starch, or fats. But it is advised that you do not feed more than 1g of starch per kg of bodyweight, per meal, or you may experience symptoms such as hypervigilance, spooky behaviour, and stereotypical behaviours such as cribbing, weaving and wind-sucking.

Feeding your horses a diet as close to their natural diet as possible is the key to maintaining not only a healthy horse, but a healthy horse's mind and behaviour, too. Wherever you can, try to allow them unlimited access to forage and hay, and make sure that your hard feed is as good as it can be.

Deficiencies can cause behavioural and performance issues, so another good tip is to have your soil tested. This way you can work out what your horses may be deficient in, because what's in the soil will go into the grass, and therefore into the horse. If you have more of an idea about what is actually going into their bodies, you stand a better chance of giving them the right things that will really give them an all-round boost.

If you keep your horses out, chances are they have access to the wild hedges that grow around so many of our fields, and you have probably turned up more than once to see them with their heads in the hedgerows, busily munching at something growing. Don't panic too much; this can actually be a really good thing! Some hedgerow plants are incredibly beneficial to horses, and I find it constantly astonishing how they tend to 'know' what the right ones are for their overall health. If your horse is constantly picking at one particular plant or other, it may be worth researching what this plant's properties are, so you can work out if your horse has a deficiency in their diet and might benefit from some supplementation.

Horses have the most amazing instincts. I am not saying that they won't (more often than you would like) get hold of something you don't want them to, but generally they are more in tune with their bodies than we are, and they will actively seek out plants that they 'know' will be good for them. I remember hearing about a horse who was diagnosed with cancer and turned away to live out his last few months in peace. The field he was in happened to be full of red clover. The horse made a beeline for this plant, which has been shown to contain isoflavones that inhibit or kill cancer cells. This horse went on to live a good few more years, healthy and happy. Coincidence? I don't think so.

A few decades ago, our pastureland was much more diverse – there would have been up to seventy different species of grass (yes, there really are that many different types) along with wild herbs and all sorts of other plant life. These days, the majority of our fields are just one or two types of grass, without the diversity that we used to see. These grasses tend to be very high in sugar and the fields are often overgrazed which further depletes the minerals in the soil. With this in mind, letting your horse pick at some other plants that may surround their fields is definitely a good thing, as they contain a vast amount of different nutrients that can benefit their bodies.

So, let's have a look at some of the hedgerow plants that can benefit your horse, plus a few that you should definitely keep them away from.

These are a few of the good ones:

Hawthorn (Crataegus)

This is a wonderful native plant, recognisable by its pointed leaves and distinctive red berries that show up in the late autumn and into winter, and it is fantastic to have in the hedgerows of your horse's field. People have used this plant for centuries to help protect against heart disease and high blood pressure, as well as a way to deal with high levels of cholesterol. Horses who seek out hawthorn can benefit from an increase in stamina, as the plant will increase coronary artery blood flow and good circulation. It also helps horses that are prone to laminitis, navicular syndrome and rheumatism. Finally, hawthorn is a great digestive aid.

Hazel (Corylus)

This tree, with its oval-shaped leaves and clusters of nuts that appear in early autumn, is another great one for your horse to nibble. The leaves provide a good foraging opportunity and are high in fibre and nutrients, while the nuts are high in protein. The leaves are said to have a beneficial effect on the digestive system, so don't be surprised if you see the horse with the ulcers reaching out for this plant. Hazel is pretty hardy and will generally spring back cheerfully even if it has been completely munched!

Dandelion (*Taraxacum officionale*)

This beautiful little weed has so many health benefits that it would be easier to list what it *isn't* good for. It is a rich source of vitamins, minerals and natural electrolytes. Dandelion has a great positive effect on the digestive system and can be used to maintain healthy bowel movements. It is also a well-known diuretic, so it can be used to help support the urinary system, too. Dandelions are also a great support to the kidneys and the liver, and a really good all-round detox for the whole body.

Cow parsley (*Anthriscus sylvestris*)

This plant is very beneficial to horses, being nutritious and very good for the digestive system. Similar to fennel, cow parsley can soothe the system and can even help to reduce flatulence. It is a good all-round immune booster for your herd, and it is even said that it can relieve stress and anxiety. This plant can also help with wound healing when taken internally. You must, however, watch out for some harmful lookalikes in the umbellifer family, particularly the poison hemlock (see below).

Red clover (*Trifolium pratense*)

This plant, with its distinctive pinkish flowers, is great for your horse's health. It is a general tonic and all-round immune system boost; it's ideal for those horses who just need a little pick-me-up. The flowers are also used as an efficient blood cleanser and they can help to improve inflammatory conditions as well. Red clover is also used as an aid to the respiratory system and it can even help with stubborn skin conditions where other treatments have failed. It is worth noting that you do not want your horse to eat too much white clover, as this can lead to a painful skin condition similar to mud fever.

Rosehip (*Rosa canina*)
Rejoice if you have a rosehip growing near the field as this plant, leaves and berries are fantastic for your horses. The berries are very high in vitamin C, which can help the body boost its immunity to certain illnesses and feeling generally run down. Rosehips contain antioxidants that can remove free radicals and help improve the immune system, plus they offer beneficial effects to the joints and can increase suppleness. Interestingly, you can feed rosehip as a preventative for those horses with an increased risk of laminitis due to polysaccharide storage myopathy (PSSM) and equine metabolic syndrome (EMS).

Cleavers (*Galium aparine*)
I always knew this plant as 'sticky willy', which used to raise a giggle from my children. As well as being great fun to stick on to people when you're out for a walk, cleavers have a great benefit to your horse's health. When they first come out in the spring, they are an excellent all-round tonic for the whole body – and horses love the taste, so they will often seek them out. They are great for supporting the lymphatic and urinary systems as they are a diuretic, so are wonderful at helping deal with swellings and inflammations. Cleavers are also very rich in silica, so they can help to strengthen the coat and the feet.

Nettles (*Urtica dioica*)
'Stingers' as we lovingly (or not so lovingly, when you unexpectedly come across a patch while poo picking!) call them, are incredibly beneficial for both horses and humans. They are an excellent cleanser for the blood and are very high in vitamins

and minerals. They also contain a surprising amount of protein and are a fantastic diuretic, so are great for treating laminitis and arthritis. Horses will eat nettles straight from the field, however much it makes us wince to watch them chewing on them, but they do prefer recently cut and wilting nettles. Nettles are also a great anti-allergy remedy. I have communicated with a large number of horses who suffer from hayfever and, without fail, the owners will say yes when I ask if their horses actively seek out nettles to eat.

Wild garlic (Allium ursinum)
We all know about the benefits of garlic. It is great for the immune system, blood cleansing and an excellent tonic for the digestive enzymes. Wild garlic is springing up around the place more and more these days, and you may be lucky enough to find it in your horse field. You will definitely notice a reduction in flies if your horse eats it, as they secrete the sulphur they absorb from the plant through their skin, which puts off irritating biting insects.

Brambles (Rubus)
Having bramble bushes around your fields is great in so many ways – not least that you can pick them to make delicious jams and puddings! Be sure to leave plenty for your horse though, they absolutely love them. And with good reason; these little berries are a powerhouse of nutrition, being filled with vitamin C and antioxidant properties. The leaves are also great, as they contain nutrients and are anti-inflammatory and antibacterial. Just keep an eye on horses' sensitive lips and tongues, as these can get spiked by the thorns and potentially cause an infection.

Many of these plants can be bought in supplement form and added to your horse's feed – as always, just keep an eye on the ingredients list, and make sure they are as pure as possible with no added ingredients. Alternatively, you can take your horse for a stroll along the lanes and encourage them to pick at these beneficial plants.

These are the bad ones:

Ragwort (*Senecio jacobaea*)

With its rosette-shaped leaves and distinctive yellow flowers, ragwort is probably familiar to most of us, given that it is present in up to 80 per cent of all horse pastures! Horses generally won't eat it when it is fresh, though you should still pull it up wherever you see it because it can sometimes get into our dried hay bales where it is much more problematic. Ragwort is more palatable when dried and, as such, the horse may eat it without even noticing. It is a 'slow burner', causing damage to the liver if ingested, meaning that by the time you notice symptoms it can be too late. Unlike some plants, its poisonous compounds are unaffected by the drying process, so it is a real concern if it ends up in your hay bales.

Sycamore (*Acer pseudoplatanus*)

A member of the Acer family, sycamore contains a substance which can kill your horse (it's hypoglycin A, in case you were interested). Although horses won't knowingly graze on the tree, they can unwittingly pick up the keys when they drop from the tree in autumn, or nibble on the sweet seedlings in the spring. It is definitely recommended that you fence your horses away from this tree, and make sure you scour the ground for leaves and keys if you have one near the field. Bear in mind that sycamore can also travel; those little helicopters can go for surprising distances. I once communicated with a horse and detected sycamore poisoning, despite the fact that there were no trees nearby. Tragically, the owners subsequently lost a three-month-old colt to sycamore poisoning shortly after.

Yew (*Taxus baccata*)

This one is an *absolute* no-no. Every single part of this tree, from the leaves to the bark, is deadly poisonous (except for a small part of the flesh of the berry), so it is definitely something that you don't want to have anywhere near horses, dogs, toddlers – or any other creature that might unwittingly ingest it. *Taxus* is so poisonous that a 1,000lb horse could be killed by ingesting as little as half a pound of the leaves, and there is no antidote beyond atropine. Keep your horses as far away from yew trees as you possibly can.

Buttercup (*Ranunculus*)

Buttercups are generally found in acidic, compacted soils (a problem for so many of us with not enough grazing to move the horses around often!) and although they are bitter-tasting, horses can pick them up on their daily grazing routes. Creeping buttercup (*Ranunculus repens*) is particularly problematic to horses as it contains glycosides and can cause poisoning. Unlike ragwort, buttercups tend to taste worse when they are dried, so finding them fresh in the pasture is more problematic than finding them in the hay, as the horses will tend to spit out the bitter dried plant.

Foxglove (*Digitalis*)

This common plant, beloved of cottage gardens, is definitely not beloved of horses. You won't generally find it growing in your fields unless you have a very natural and diverse pasture, but it is worth watching out for if you ride past people's gardens. As with many poisonous plants horses won't actively seek it out, but do watch out for a sneaky mouthful plucked while you're out and about, or dried in your hay bales, as even a small amount can cause fatal problems due to the cardioactive steroids, including digitoxin and digoxin. This one can be treated with some success, if a vet is called in quickly enough.

Privet (*Ligustrum*)
A very popular hedging plant, privet can be found just about everywhere – it is evergreen and makes a great hedge and screen. It is not great for horses, though. They cannot digest it and it causes severe gastrointestinal distress – ingestion of privet can lead to death within forty-eight hours unless you know your horse ate it and you can bring in a vet very quickly.

Rhododendron (*Rhododendron*)
This is a non-native plant that is very popular as a hedging plant as it grows quickly and is hard to get rid of. Rhododendron is highly poisonous to horses because of the cardiac glycosides, but luckily, they are very unlikely to eat it even if it borders their fields, because it has an unpleasant taste. Do watch out for this plant being close to your horse's field if grazing is very sparse, however, as they may reach for it out of desperation for something green.

Oak (*Quercus*)
Another common tree that grows in hedgerows and around our fields is oak, which can cause problems for horses – especially those who are already immune-compromised or otherwise weak. Unlike many of the other poisonous plants, horses actually enjoy eating oak leaves and acorns, but ingesting them can cause digestive problems and discomfort. Try to keep your horse away from oak trees if you possibly can.

Bracken (*Pteridium*)
This is probably not going to be too much of a problem in your horse's field, as bracken tends to grow on well-drained moorland, but it's worth keeping an eye out for when you are out riding. Horses will generally avoid bracken and it is not as toxic as some others in this list, but eating it repeatedly over a long period of time can prove fatal.

Hemlock (*Conium maculatum*)

Hemlock, like many others in the same family, is deadly poisonous to just about everything. Every part of the plant is toxic, and this one can kill a horse within two hours. They tend not to graze it, because it smells horrible and we assume that it also tastes nasty, but as with other plants, it can be a big problem if it ends up dried in the hay, where it will not be as noticeable. It looks very similar to cow parsley, but hemlock has distinctive purple patches on the stem. Avoid this one at all costs.

I like to encourage us to be as natural as possible with the countryside, and certainly don't advocate destroying flora as it is, in many cases, a food source and a habitat for many different species. However, if you have any of these plants in your locality, keep your horses fenced off from them to avoid any potential disasters.

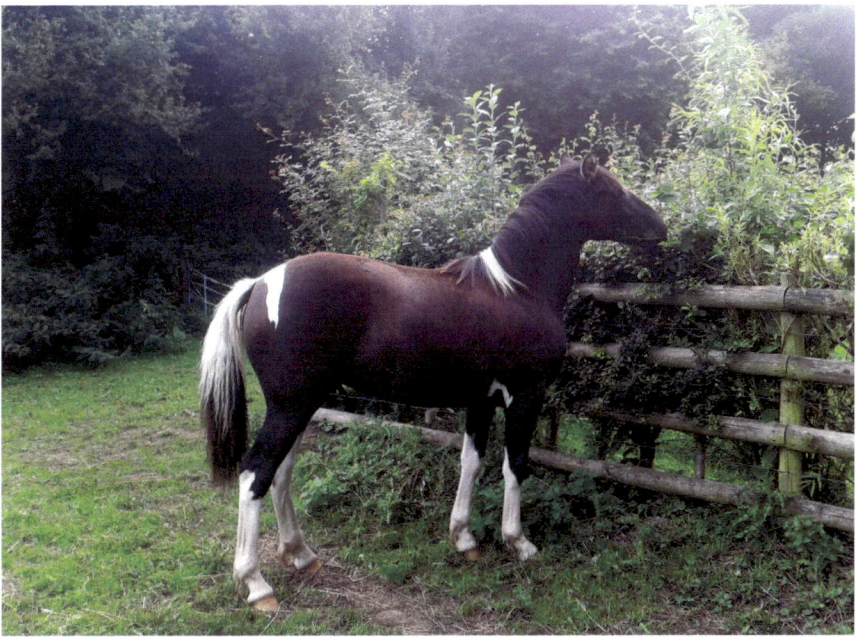

Eating plants from the hedgerows can be very beneficial to your horse. (Faith Hancock)

It can be tricky to work out what to feed your horses for the best. Obviously, keeping things as natural as possible is the ideal, as is feeding your horse the appropriate diet for their workload and body type. I always encourage allowing horses to pick at what they like – within reason, of course – as, unlike us, they have an innate sense of what is good for them. Definitely look up the hedgerow plants they seem to go for the most. As long as you are sure none of them are on the 'bad list', it can be a really useful insight into what your horse needs in their diet.

Many horses, especially if they are rescues or have had a poor start, can get anxious about food. There are a great many horses that I have spoken to who have confessed that their aggression around food stems from worrying that they won't have enough, especially if they have been kept short in the past.

Try to ensure that they are not kept hungry – although you may have to explain to that fat little native pony that being allowed to eat as much as his thoroughbred companion will cause him health issues! Make sure there is always access to grass and/or hay, as the roughage will help their digestion and allow them to feel relaxed and comfortable.

One final note about food – boredom can also be a factor in over-eating or being pushy about food. If your horses stay in, make sure they have small-holed hay nets that allow them to eat, but not as fast. Put a few toys around the place and visit very often, to keep them happy and to prevent the dreaded boredom-eating.

6

FEET

Let's face it, it really is no good having a horse that has trouble with its feet, is it? I mean, it's not much fun for either of you! Strong, healthy hooves that never go lame, never throw an abscess, never lose a shoe – that's the dream, isn't it? And just imagine how happy we'd all be without laminitis!

Every single horse has distinctive feet; some breeds' hooves are naturally stronger than others, and horses in different types of work and living conditions will exhibit different feet. Apart from a good farrier, good nutrition and good living conditions – what else do you need to know?

Horses' feet can be something of a tricky subject – there are many people who swear by regular shoeing, and equally as many who swear by barefoot. Obviously, it's down to personal preference, but also, it's about trying to do the best for your horse – this is what we all strive for, every single day. There are myriad arguments on both sides, on the benefits of shoeing versus barefoot and I'll tell you right now that I'm not going to get into it, except to say some horses do better barefoot, some are better shod.

Aside from whether or not your horse is shod, there are some incredible things to learn about their feet. It is pretty easy to spot when there's a stone stuck in a hoof and also to know the telltale

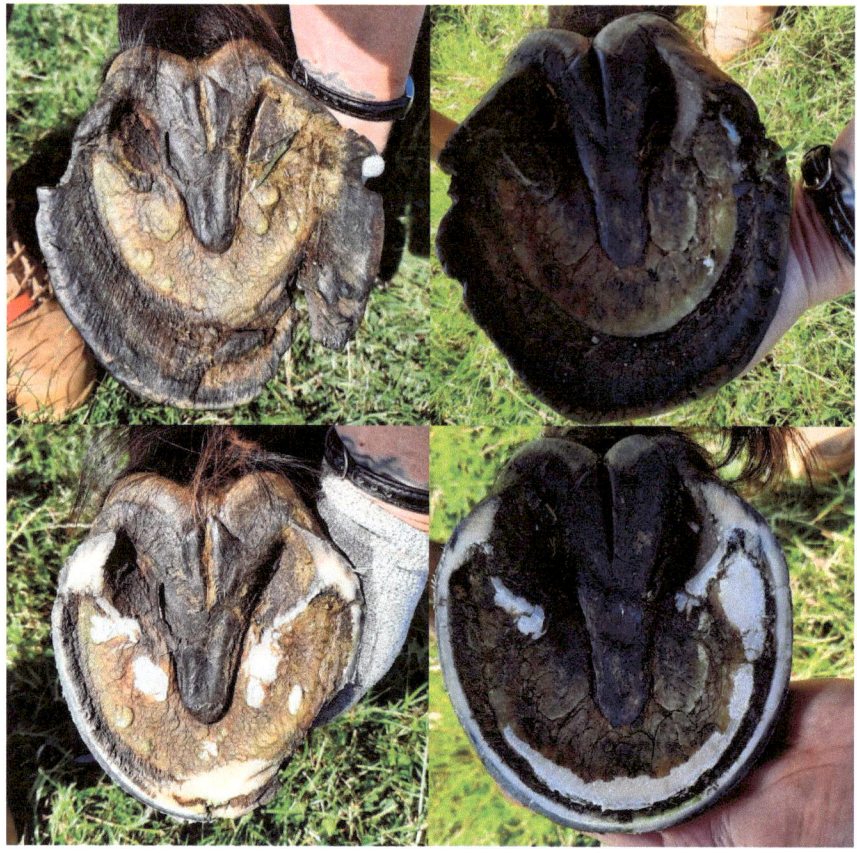

A progression from an overgrown hoof to a well-trimmed hoof. (Anna Curtis)

signs of an abscess forming, but what about the trickier parts of horses' hooves that we cannot necessarily see? What can we do to make our horses' feet stronger? To shoe or not to shoe?

Obviously in the wild, horses don't wear shoes. Horses are designed to roam around for hours at a time, wearing down the edges of their feet as they get longer on their natural terrain. Well, mustangs and others who live in dry arid conditions do anyway. Those that live in wetter, marshy climates, like the Camargues of France, will tend to grow rather long hooves that chip off in large chunks, rather than wearing down into the smooth half-moon shape that we all know and love from old cowboy movies.

Feet

The problem comes, as it so often does, when we domesticate them and try to get them to fit in with our lifestyles. Evidence of horses being shod has been found as far back as 400 BC; the materials tended to be rawhide, leather and plants. These were used both as protection for the hoof and as a means of soothing existing injuries.

Metal horseshoes came much later and historians and archaeologists tend to argue about the origins of these. It is safe to say, though, that by the time of the Industrial Revolution the horseshoe business had really started to take off.

There are both advantages and disadvantages to being barefoot, in the same way that there are to being shod. A shod horse is often more comfortable on rough ground than a barefoot one, especially if that horse has naturally sensitive feet. A barefoot horse can actually grow stronger feet as a result of being barefoot, as the hoof will respond to its environment. Conversely, a horse that is constantly in shoes can develop more sensitive soles, due to them never really being in contact with the ground. Shoes can lift the foot, which is good for those with weaker feet.

As you can see, it's almost as controversial as 'Should I bottle feed or breastfeed?' So, I'm really not going to get into a debate – you just have to do the right thing for your horse. I'm sure you already do! As long as your horse's feet are regularly trimmed and maintained by a good farrier, or if you take and pass one of the many trimming courses out there and learn how to do it yourself; both are equally valid – then you are doing the right thing.

A wonderful equine podiatrist I know describes the hoof as 'the canary in the coal mine', because you can see in a hoof what has happened to a body. In a similar way to humans growing stress ridges or discolourations on their nails due to trauma or nutritional deficiency, many of a horse's problems show up in their hooves.

The healthiest horse will have the healthiest hooves. In the same way that gut issues show up if something is lacking in the diet, feet can reveal things that are not ideal in the horse's general health. If the horse has adequate food, accommodation and exercise, or at the very least *two* of those things, they will generally be pretty healthy and their feet should be good, too. However, if fewer than two of these factors are in place then problems will start to show up in the feet.

For example, if there is inflammation (illness, stress or some other trauma) anywhere in the body, it will show up in the hooves in the form of bruises, or in a raised digital pulse. Laminitis, one of the most common ailments that affects our horses, can be detected by feeling the digital pulse – if a raised pulse is present in all four hooves, you may be looking at a case of laminitis. If a raised pulse is only showing in one hoof, it is generally a more localised reaction somewhere else in the body.

There are way too many variables to be able to say, 'This is what you must do to ensure your horse has healthy feet, all the time, and never has any problems!' So, I'm not going to do that. Instead, we're just going to look at a few of the things that I know can affect the health of the hoof and therefore the health of the entire horse.

Diet

I have already said quite a lot about diet, haven't I? Sorry, but I've got to bring it into hoof health, too. Thankfully, horse feed is getting better. In times gone by no one really knew about the inflammatory effects of many of the ingredients and the quality was definitely substandard – and covered with molasses, to make it palatable, which added to the problems. However, many horses today are nutritionally deficient – and that's not necessarily your fault. Feeds that are contaminated with pesticides can be harmful, and the use of cheap oils as lubricants can also cause a great deal of health problems.

Even the hay, lovingly bought at great expense from a local farm, can change in quality depending on where it was harvested and at what time of year. I agree, it's a nightmare to get it right. But once you do, you will notice not only a change in your horse's hoof health, but also in their behaviour.

Diet is also one of the biggest factors in laminitis. There are a number of different types of laminitis, but excessive consumption of sugar or starch is a big factor in all of them. You don't really need a better excuse to allow your horse the most natural diet possible, do you? Of course, some horses will be prone to the condition anyway, due to a previous experience, but you can just do the best you can – and get a great farrier.

Accommodation

Where and how the horse is kept plays a huge part in the health of a hoof, as do food, exercise and general health. Horses' feet are sensitive to their surroundings, as I said with my comparison of mustangs and Camargues, so it makes sense that your horse's feet will reflect their environment.

For example, if your horse is barefoot and lives in a hard, dry field on top of a hill, you may notice sand cracks, chips and the odd bit of bruising. If you keep your horse shod and in deep litter, you may experience issues with pathogens and bacteria, as damp conditions do soften the foot.

Remember that the time of year can also affect the feet; when it tends to be wetter and muddier in the winter months, even a stabled horse is likely to get soggy while riding. This can soften the sole, and you can start to see more fungal infections. The hot, dry summer months may show up more cracks and chips – and an artificial sole can actually grow over the hoof bed, as it doesn't naturally exfoliate in the hotter months.

Keeping an eye on your horse's hooves is not only a necessary part of owning a horse and maintaining their fitness, but it can also be a great way to keep an eye on the health of their entire body – and changing things up if it's necessary.

Exercise

This is more than a means of keeping your horse fit enough for competitions, or able to take you on long pleasure rides every weekend – exercising a horse, as I'm sure you know, is really good for them. The number of horses I come across who are grumpy because they are bored and under-stimulated is just crazy. I know it can be very hard to find the time, or the resources to exercise a horse as much as they might need, but you will notice a very positive change in hoof health if you do.

Exercise is a great way to open up the lungs, get the blood coursing, the lymphatic system draining, the sweat going to excrete the toxins. Also, it's a good way of converting energy in the form of food into muscle. A horse can weigh the same in muscle and fat, but the muscle version will be healthier – not least because there will be no layers of fat around the internal organs, and the fat can carry toxins.

If your horse is enjoying an appropriate level of exercise suitable for their breed and their type – whether this is just blasting around the field a few times a day, or going on four-hour hacks – you will notice the health of their feet as well as the rest of their body improving.

Stress

Horses are naturally prey animals, and as such they can be pretty actively attuned to any little thing that might be a threat (as you probably know, if you've had one of those horses who was convinced that the hosepipe was a venomous snake that was trying to kill them!). Therefore, is it too far-fetched to expect them not to be extremely susceptible to things like stress? It's all very well for us to move them around the countryside to go to shows, or to take their field mate out for a hack – we know we're all coming back home at the end of the day, right? Horses don't necessarily know that – or rather, they don't necessarily *think* that.

Horses' reactions to stress can sometimes show up in their hooves in the form of growth rings. Generally, if they are wider at the toe than at the base of the hoof, this indicates some inflammation in the body. If they are straight from heel to toe, it shows a sudden change in diet. On very rare occasions, a horse can show an 'event fracture', which is a crack all the way around the hoof, on all four hooves, because the growth of the hoof has been stopped in its tracks because of a traumatic event. Similar to humans, who get lines or ridges on their fingernails during times of stress, or the nails stop growing completely, horses will show similar stress reactions in their hooves. My equine podiatrist tells a story of one horse she had seen who had shown this, and she asked his owner what had happened around four months previously, which was around the timescale of the event fracture based on the rate of hoof growth. The owner thought for a while then replied, 'His companion was put down around then ...' and it all became clear. This horse was showing the trauma he had suffered, in a way that couldn't be argued with – horses feel stress and trauma, too, and it can show up in their bodies – most noticeably in their feet.

Horses' hooves are literally the bedrock of all they are, so make sure you look after them as well as you possibly can. If you can't work it out yourself, get a really good farrier. When farriers trim our horses' feet, they are all aiming for that lovely half-moon shape, a good strong sole and a healthy frog – whether or not your horse is shod, these are the foundations of a good healthy foot that can see you and your horse over many miles. A farrier is trying to replicate the miles of wear and tear that a horse would receive in six weeks in the wild, in one half-hour session trimming those toes. Bear this in mind, the next time your wild horse decides to lean their entire weight on them or casually wave a back leg in the direction of their face!

If you're lucky, you have a great farrier who is kind and sensitive with your horses, and who achieves the right trim and the right shoeing schedule for you. Bonus points if they know everything there is to know about feet and can use these 'little canaries' to help you understand more about your horse's general health.

7

ON THE TRACKS

Where we keep our horses can have a drastic effect on their well-being, both mentally and physically. Horses in the wild tend to roam for long distances in search of food or water – though they generally have a territory that they roughly stick to. Horses that

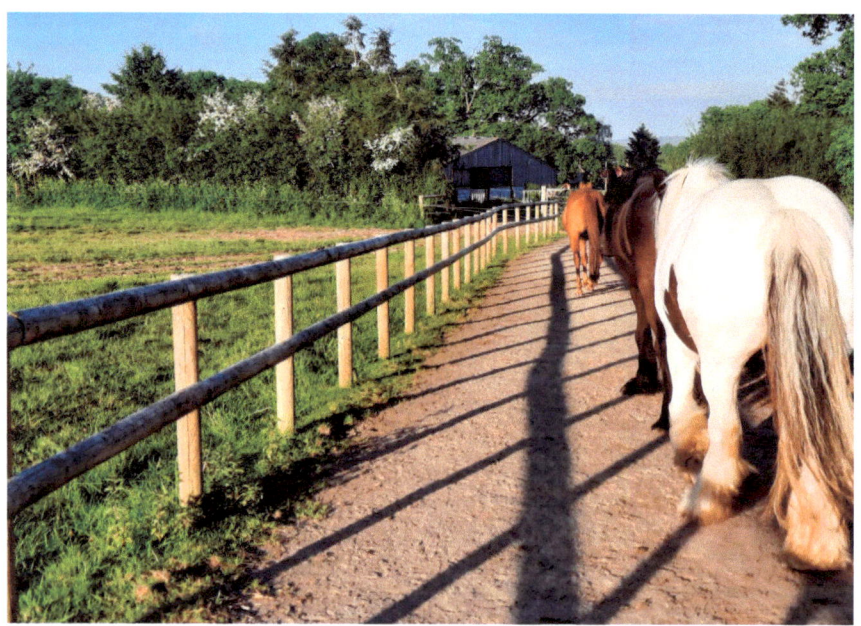

A track system can encourage exercise and natural ways of foraging. (Anna Curtis)

we keep as riding horses, therapy animals, eventers or even pets, don't have this luxury.

Obviously, the most important thing is that your horse's accommodation is safe and secure. They need to be kept safe from dangers such as traffic, people, some types of plants, and even themselves (you'll know what I mean if you have one of those who can injure themselves by just looking at barbed wire!). They also need stimulation, a good bond with other horses, decent food and free access to water.

If you have an outside space then this is ideal. Horses are not designed to live indoors. However, many horses need to be kept in as that is what they are used to, and putting them straight out twenty-four hours a day, seven days a week, can cause them a lot of problems – but the ones who *do* live out constantly, tend to develop thick coats and thick skins, and can handle even the worst of the weather.

I have no problem with stabling and, in fact, I kept Ranger stabled with a fairly strict routine – without this I wouldn't have been able to catch him, ever! If stabling is how you keep your horses then that's absolutely fine; if it works for you and your horses then that's fantastic. But there is no denying that it is not the most natural way to keep horses – and is not generally the way that they themselves would choose to be kept. There is so much information out there these days on the best ways to keep our horses, some that may seem radical when you first learn about them, and a great deal of information that we can use to support our horses to be as healthy and happy as they possibly can be.

Of course, every horse is different – some love a warm, cosy barn, others just want to be out every day of the year no matter what the weather. I have spoken to many horses who have issues with their accommodation – some just don't like to be kept in *at all*, while others love the feeling of being pampered and warm that comes with a stabled life. Interestingly, I once spoke to a horse whose owner was considering a track system and had sat in his stable while going through her plans. Her horse told me that he 'loved the patch of sand' that she was planning, while she couldn't believe that he had even heard her talk about it or had his own opinions on it! (He now lives out on said track system and his owner reports that he loves it, and never wants to come in!)

In the middle of an English winter, or even in the spring and summer if we're honest, our fields can end up looking a lot like a swamp. It's horrible to look outside and see our friends standing hock-deep in mud! The instinct is to bring them inside, where they're warm and cosy and to keep the worst of the weather off them. If you do not have access to inside accommodation and your horses live out all year, winter can look and feel pretty bleak. But, constant stabling is not necessarily what your horse wants.

Horses are not like us; they don't tend to scamper indoors at the first sight of rain and many don't even seem to feel the cold at all. I can't count the number of days I have visited horses and seen their manes and whiskers adorned with ice crystals. Yes, the amount of mud and rain can get them down and you will often find them standing under trees for shelter. But a great many of them will ignore a barn or a stable, even if the option is open to them.

Many of my clients report that their horses, despite the lovely dry, warm field shelter or the cosy stable, much prefer being out all day. Some horses I know just don't like being in stables. Many do, of course, but others are not suited to this environment. Being constantly stabled and having a strict routine can cause horses quite a lot of problems. Feeding at the same time every day can leave them with anxiety issues – especially if the car won't start and you are half an hour late. They can often be more aggressive around food, because they know it is not constantly available to them, so they feel they have to really make the most of it as soon as any sign of it appears. Boredom-based problems such as wind-sucking and crib biting can come from feeling 'cooped up'.

A horse who is stabled for long periods of the day will not only get bored, but they can also start to display health issues. Horses have no muscles in their legs from the knee down, so they rely on the flow of the blood caused by moving around to keep the circulatory and lymphatic systems functioning as they should. Ever wondered why your horse's legs swell when they are standing in the stable for too long?

I'm not saying, 'Don't stable your horse, ever!' It's really nice to tuck them up into bed with a warm feed and a nice rug, isn't it? I'm just saying that, although it is the way that most of us have been brought up to keep our horses, there are definitely better ways.

If you are looking for a really good way of keeping your horses, so that they are as natural and as happy as they can possibly be, then you may want to look into a track system. The track system as we know it today was pioneered by a man called Jamie Jackson, an American farrier.

He was noticing so many chronic issues with horses' feet that he took himself off to study the wild mustangs in their natural environment and noted that horses will walk on well-designated paths, sometimes for up to 30km a day. Their feet were pretty perfect, and their way of life was clearly responsible for this, as these horses were completely wild and had never been trimmed or shod. Interestingly, they also had far fewer – if any – metabolic issues, and none would suffer from ulcers, laminitis or Cushing's disease.

Track system

The track system is less about field management and feeding (though it is also very helpful with these things, too) than keeping horses in as natural a way as possible and allowing them to move around freely. Keeping horses in stables, or on very small patches of land, often with individual turnout, is not actually the best thing for them. A track system is widely hailed as the absolute best living situation for horses with health problems, excessive weight, or foot issues.

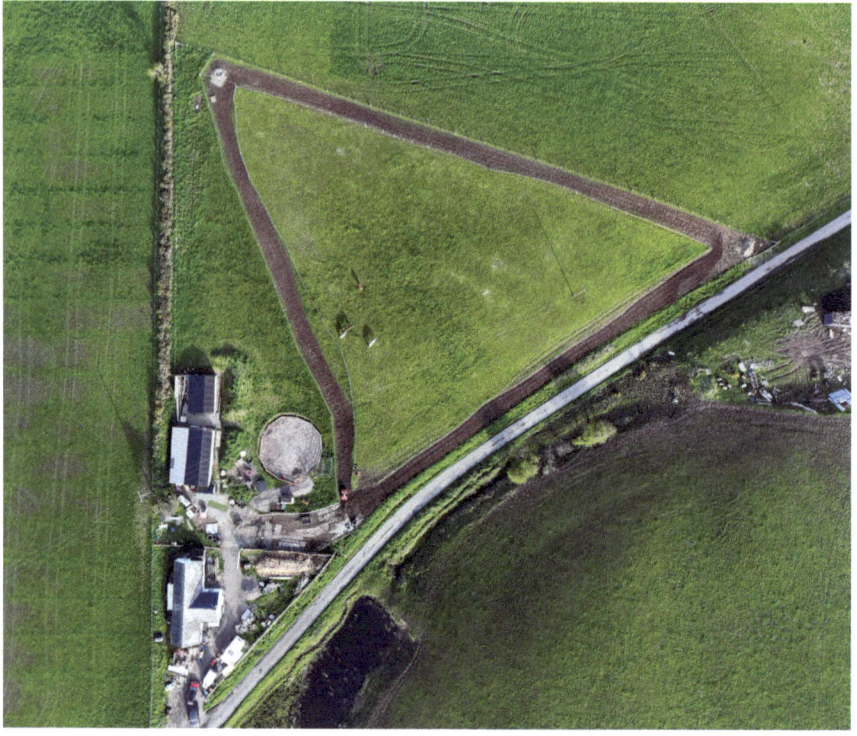

Tracks are pretty big from the air! (Dr John Shephard)

If you think about where horses first originated from – the northern hemisphere and the steppes of Eurasia – they would not have had huge fields full of gleaming green grass. They had rough terrain, rough forage – and, some would say, rough lives, though that is a view coloured by how we picture keeping horses today.

The way that they evolved meant that they would be constantly moving and always in their herd environments, with all the different family and social connections that this entails. Remember that horses are herd animals, and being without companions can make them miserable. If you think about it, we actually interact with our horses very little. We have work, busy lives and families, so the time that we spend with our horses probably only amounts to a few hours a day (unless you're lucky enough to have them living right outside your door). What do you think your horse is doing for the rest of the time, when you are not there?

Allowing horses to move around freely is incredibly good for them. Not only will you see less incidences of weight gain and the issues that come with this, but the feet will be generally healthier – plus the problems that are associated with behavioural issues will be considerably lower. Most people who use a track system report that their horses are more chilled out, happier, and are able to relax into their natural ways of being – with each other, and with their owners.

Track systems are generally a long track (the clue is in the name!), which is often circular, or in whatever other pattern that you want to create. The food is ideally situated as far away from the water as possible, so the horses have to move between the two, thus getting their daily steps in.

Some track systems use mud mats – these are great because they are movable (unless they get buried beneath layers of mud) and they stop the mud from getting too deep and unmanageable. Other systems use a hardcore base, which is trying to mimic the natural environment of the horse. You should have different areas with different textures – for example, one area that is rocky and stony; another that has sand for them to roll and sleep; maybe another that is allowed to just be muddy – because who doesn't love to spend hours grooming or getting the hosepipe out?

Ideally, you should be feeding hay constantly. Yes, this is expensive, but if you compare a hay bill with a hefty vet's bill then I'm sure you'll see the difference! By placing hay all around the track at different intervals, your horses will be able to move around, picking their favourite bits out of each pile as they go, then going back to eventually finish it all off.

You can add various enrichment activities to the track system to keep your horses engaged and happy, but if they are mooching around with their herd members in a natural environment, you will probably find that they don't have as much need for toys and other things that we use to keep them engaged.

Strip grazing

If you don't want to keep your horses stabled but you don't have the space or inclination for a track system, strip grazing is another good option. This is a great system for both limiting the amount of grass your horses get in the summer, and for saving it for the winter. It generally involves quite a lot of electric tape, which is no one's favourite fencing system, but it can be very beneficial to both the horses and the land itself – it stops the horses overgrazing and getting the health issues that come with this, plus it gives the land a break from overgrazing and poaching.

If you have the space, you should separate a large area off in the spring or summer, then rest this area completely and leave the horses off it until the winter. The longer grass, although it gives us laminitis vibes to just look at, contains far fewer sugars than the shorter, sweeter grass, so you shouldn't have to worry too much about letting them out on it when the grazing is short in the winter.

You can move the fence little and often; just a few feet along the whole strip every couple of days will allow for some happy foraging – though you will almost certainly find them grazing right at the edges of the fence, staring longingly at the grass beyond! This is a fairly labour-intensive way of grazing, as you will have to be moving that fence a few times a week to allow grazing on the new grass, but it is very good for your horses and your fields.

Another downside to strip grazing is that the horses can get so excited about the new grass, that they'll just eat everything in sight as soon as you move the fence, so you will have to be extra vigilant for harmful plants like ragwort. They can (and almost certainly will) trample all over the new section you have just released, which can seem a little counterintuitive, but the grass will bounce back, and in most cases more quickly than if it is left to be freely grazed throughout the year, with the poaching and compaction that goes with this.

Rotation

This is a great option if you have a few fields or a large patch of land, and it can mean that you have to use less temporary fencing. (I can hear those of us who shudder at the sight of poly posts and tape breathing a sigh of relief from here!)

Basically, this involves letting the horses out into one field and just leaving them to it, while the other areas rest and regrow. It works pretty well, even in the winter when everything is poached, or the summer when it looks as dry and arid as a desert – you may have to still feed hay, but as this is good for them and takes longer to eat than all the grass, it's no big deal really.

As with the strip grazing method, you might be worried about letting the horses loose onto knee-length grass – but remember, it is actually more dangerous for them when it is very short, as there are far more sugars present in the short grass than the long. It will almost certainly stay long for a while after they have been let loose onto it, as they will pick at the best bits, and come back for the rest once their favourite bits have been eaten.

Sadly, the type of grass and the conditions that we have in this country are just not what horses have evolved to eat or to live in. They are designed to wander for miles and miles on hard ground, picking at whatever forage they can find – and for thousands of years this is just what they did. They survived quite well without stables, leg bandages and foot trimming, thank you very much!

But we have to work with what we've got, and in this country that is, sadly, mainly damp, wet conditions and fields full of high-sugar rye grass. Our horses have to deal with many health issues because of these conditions, and we do what we can to minimise the impact of this on them, but there is only so much we can do, as the majority of us are not millionaires.

We don't all have the luxury of our own fields and track systems; some of us are bound by livery yard rules, stabling, or footpaths through our fields. I get it, I really do, and we all have to make the most of what we've got. But, making steps towards keeping your horses as naturally as possible – in a herd, with plenty of space to roam about and be horses, plenty of natural roughage to support the guts, and a hard, dry ground to support the feet – will make life infinitely better for both them and for you.

8

BEHAVIOURAL ISSUES

Now, it's all very well to say that your horse is acting out because he or she is in pain, or is being fed the wrong type of food, or has foot problems. We can sort these things, and obviously we all want to fix any issues as quickly as we can, to improve the health and well-being of our beloved friends.

But what about if you've had everything checked out, you know it's not a physical issue, and they're *still* just unpleasant to be around? The tack has been checked; the whole body treated for pain and injury; their needs are all completely met and you treat them with sensitivity and love – and yet they still insist on charging you in the field, refusing to be caught, or rearing suddenly halfway through a ride. This may well make you feel that there is no reason for their behaviour.

Let me tell you, no horse – or child, for that matter – is *just* an unpleasant being. There's always a reason for it. Once you find the reason, you can delve down into the unwanted behaviour, find out why it is happening, and take steps towards getting it to improve. I do relate horses to children a lot, don't I? This is because, when you look at it, they are pretty similar:

They don't have the same abilities to communicate as a grown-up, well-adjusted adult.

They lack impulse control.
They tend to express themselves very dramatically if something is happening that they don't like.
Their behaviour can be dangerous.
And they are often hugely misunderstood.

For many years, children and horses have been treated as if they don't have thoughts and feelings at all; that they are only here as an afterthought to our own, incredibly important, lives. The attitude has been that they should be punished for having an opinion, and if they don't fit in with our lifestyles then they must be 'broken' in order to do so. Tantrums are a sign of 'naughtiness' and should be punished. Daydreaming should be punished. Natural behaviours should be punished until they fit in with our ideal of a society.

Because of this attitude, in times gone by, children have grown up with countless mental health issues, and horses have been treated like commodities, easily picked up and thrown away when they were used up – or shot needlessly because they were not being 'heard'.

Thankfully these days, we are edging towards a more natural, gentle and respectful way of treating children – and horses. It is no longer acceptable to simply say a child is being naughty and sending them to the time-out corner; we are now starting to realise that any sort of acting out is a need that is not being met. We are beginning to see a great deal of nuance in the different personalities and behaviours, and learning to accept them as they are.

It is exactly the same with our horses. Learning to understand them, to treat them with respect and love, acknowledging that they are also sentient beings with thoughts, feelings and a totally individual personality – all this is working to improve our relationships, our riding careers and our general understanding.

If a horse who categorically has no pain, inflammation or illness anywhere in his body is *still* being unpleasant, we have to look

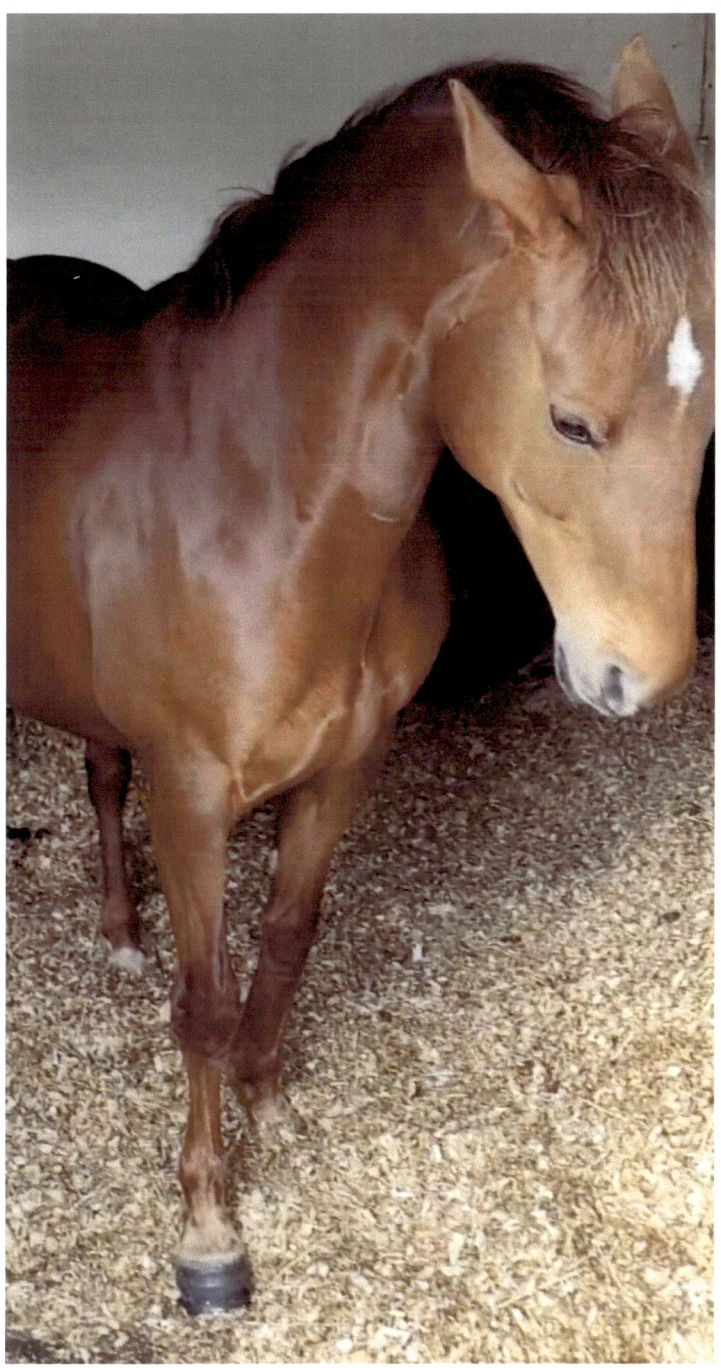

What to do when they're grumpy for no reason? (Hannah Tomo)

for other reasons for this behaviour. Thankfully, there are many different things you can look into – and have a go at fixing – which may well take great steps to improving the behaviour.

Are they bored? Are they overstimulated? Do they dislike their accommodation? How is their relationship with the rest of their herd – in fact, do they even *have* a herd? Did they experience a lot of stress and trauma in a previous home? Have they been kept short of food? Do they even trust people at all, if they have suffered earlier trauma?

All these factors will have an effect on how your horse is behaving. Yes, some of the behaviour is not enjoyable – just like a toddler having a meltdown in the supermarket aisle, tantrum behaviour in your horse is definitely something to be avoided! As you would hopefully do with a toddler, you would find out what is causing the horse's behaviour, then work out how you can improve it in the future.

Obviously if it is a non-negotiable thing such as safety, health or hygiene then you do it anyway, with both toddlers and horses. Your horse *needs* to see the vet, no matter how much they dislike it. There may be no other option than to keep them next to that gelding they hate. They cannot throw a tantrum on the main road, if it can possibly be avoided. These are just a few examples.

But, if there is a way to understand the behaviour better, empathise with the big feelings and work around the issue together, you will find that you are building a relationship based on respect and trust, rather than on fear and anger. You will almost certainly find that with this approach, your horse actually manages to work through the unwanted behaviour, rather than you both sweeping it under the rug and getting on with it in the hope that it'll go away by itself (spoiler alert – it probably won't).

Now, I don't go in for owner-shaming any more than I do for horse-shaming. But the fact is, however hard it may be to hear, that *you* just might be a factor in your horse's behavioural issues. Hear me out! I'm not saying that you are causing your horse to act in the way that they do, but horses are incredibly sensitive creatures.

If you are going into the yard or the field with a mindset, consciously or subconsciously, that your horse is going to misbehave, then the chances are they will. If you are entering their space with some leftover anger or frustration from the last time they did a horrible thing, they might just pick up on that and repeat the behaviour. If your head is not firmly focused on them, and what you are going to do, they may realise that and act out accordingly.

It is very important to remember that horses are prey animals. They look to their herd to protect them and keep them safe, which is why if one herd member is frightened or flighty, they will instantly perceive a threat, and go on the defensive. You are a herd member, too, remember that! If these incredibly sensitive animals pick up on the fact that you are nervous or scared, they will think that there is something to be scared of.

Your horse may well have exhibited some behaviour that has frightened you – in fact, I'd struggle to think of any horse owner who has not been scared by something their horse has done, at some point during their time together – but it is important to try and reduce that fear. Your horse will know if you are feeling scared, which in turn makes them feel scared, which can lead to unwanted behaviour.

A horse is rarely mean, they just react to an action (and it may have taken time for it to have got to this point) and in the absence of a voice, email or text, this is their only way of expressing when they aren't happy or feel unsafe to be touched. Something may have spooked your horse, something that you dismissed as not really being anything, but in their minds, it is as big and scary as that time a tiger (aka a plastic bag!) tried to jump out of the fence and eat them.

Horses have a quasi-photographic memory, meaning that they can remember places, faces, and even different expressions.

They can recall that time your face was like thunder when you discovered them helping themselves to the contents of their feed bin, or when you shouted at them for pushing a herd member off the hay pile. Practising keeping your energy calm and relaxed when you interact with them will help, I promise.

As with us, horses have people that they like and those that they don't. You may have a horse who anyone can ride, or you may be an owner like so many whose horses will only tolerate them. Who can be surprised? If you don't know someone, or you take a disliking to them for whatever reason, you are not going to play nicely with them. So often, I talk to a horse and find out that they really love their owner – this is one of the best parts of my job; helping the partnership to understand that 'bad' behaviour is not a result of our horses not liking us, which is an immense relief to many horse owners.

If your horse is fine with you but acts out with other people, just know that this is completely normal. If you are the sort of person who treats your horse with kindness and respect, and you have a good bond, can you really be surprised if they object when a stranger (to them) decides to get on and then starts trying to make them do things? I once communicated with a horse who put a very famous (naming no names) rider through a set of poles, not once or twice but three times, because she didn't like the way he was riding her. It's not too surprising, when you think about it.

We need to remember to treat our horses with respect. This includes, but is not limited to saying 'please', 'thank you', 'will you?', 'could you?' I'm not saying that you should let them run roughshod over you, but as your granny probably used to say, 'A little politeness goes a long way.' Saying 'thank you' is an important one – you will very rarely see a top eventer finishing a round without giving the horse a pat or a cuddle, even if everything went wrong and they ate dirt or smashed through five jumps before refusing to go on. This is the kind of respectful, loving working relationship we should all be striving for – whether you are a horse parent of some field ornaments, or you are aiming for the top heights of dressage fame. They are trying really hard for you, so make sure they are acknowledged for this – even if they don't get it right first time.

Horses are equally as clever, equally as knowing, and *at least* as emotionally intelligent as humans – and in some cases they are more so. They are incredibly forgiving; I see this especially in my job, as I can pick up on how much pain a horse may be in, but they are still trying to do their work and give their all. They give us warnings – making faces while we're doing up the girth of *that* particular saddle, or resisting *that* particular transition – and this is invariably because of pain or discomfort in the body. They are, as you probably already know, extremely sensitive, and totally individual. You may have two horses who like or dislike the same things, but their reactions to these things will be totally different, based on their individual personalities.

There are a few generalised basic personality types in horses – obviously, each one will vary from horse to horse, but they do seem to fit into a rough selection: confident and extroverted; unconfident but extroverted; confident and introverted; and introverted plus unconfident. Obviously, these traits can be more or less noticeable, depending on the health of the horse, the herd dynamic, the general circumstances, and what you are asking of your horse, but they generally fit into one of these four boxes … as do you.

Are you a confident extrovert struggling with a horse that is shy and timid? Or do you feel steamrollered by your extroverted, confident horse when you wanted to take things slowly and calmly? These can be issues for all of us with our horses (and with some people we know). Their personalities can have a big effect on your daily lives together, and although this should go without saying, it has taken quite a long time for people to realise that horses are 'individuals', too, with their own personalities, their likes and dislikes, and their own characteristics.

It is well worth noting down your own characteristics and those of your horse, to ensure that you are working together well and not butting heads. It might be an idea to ask a friend or family member to do this for you, as we aren't always the best at working out who and what we are ourselves.

Now ask yourself, what is it about your horse that first attracted you? What are they doing that goes against your innermost personality? What does your horse seem to need that they are not getting from you? How can you adjust your demands of your horse to accommodate their innate personality and start really achieving in your partnership together?

I have only met one or two horses in the whole time I have been doing this job, who were what I would call 'truly bad apples'. The vast majority, hundreds and thousands of them, are acting out because of pain or distress. Instead of just writing them off as that nuisance in the field, try to look a little deeper. What's *really* going on with them? Get all the extra help you can – have the tack fitted; have the physical therapy; have the teeth done; check the diet. You will almost certainly find that your horse, and your relationship with them, improves no end.

I, for one, am so grateful to be seeing the change in mindset that is going on these days, where we are far more aware and respectful of our fellow creatures, and I think it is improving life for all of us – the two legged as well as the four legged.

9

WHAT TO WEAR

If your horse is ridden, the chances are you will have spent a great deal of time and money researching what sort of tack they should be in. Hopefully you will have got a saddle fitter out, and done some research on what the best type of tack there is out there for your horse, or maybe you have stuck with the same old kit simply because it comes from a brand you like and trust, which has served you well in the past.

However, tack can cause a lot of problems for our horses. Just imagine if you had to go to work every day, wearing something that was too small, or too big, or rubbed and chafed in uncomfortable places that you couldn't fix by yourself. I doubt you'd be at your most productive and happy, would you? In fact, you may come to dread a job that you had previously loved, because you had to wear something that was uncomfortable for you.

Can you guess what I'm going to say? Yes. Your horse is exactly the same. They can be the happiest, calmest, most gentle dope-on-a-rope on the ground, but as soon as you get that saddle out they start pinning their ears back and giving you the murderous side-eye. This is your horse trying to tell you something.

If you cannot fix the problem, your horse is going to carry on showing you that they are not comfortable in the only way they

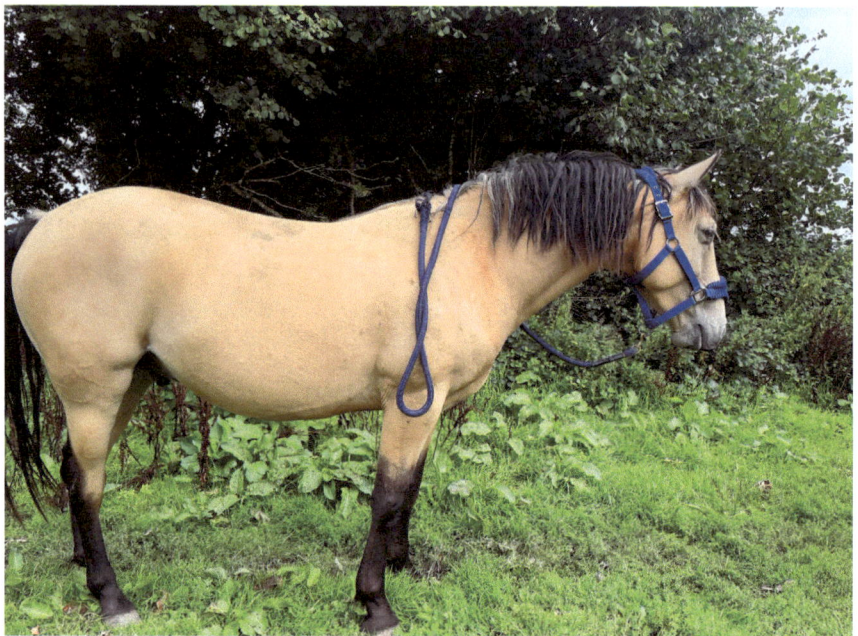

'I have a whole wardrobe, and I still have nothing to wear!' (Kaia Ede)

know how – by trying to get rid of the discomfort. If this gets rid of you, too, then this is a necessary side effect, in their mind! I know this is not much comfort for you as you sail through the air and land face first yet again, but it should be a relief to you to know that there is a lot you can do about this problem.

Your first port of call should be a professional tack fitter who can help you make sure that your saddle is the right fit, and that it is not pinching or rubbing your horse.

Saddles can be adjusted via several methods, one being changeable gullet bars. This adjustment only changes the width of the saddle to certain sizes, so if the horse changes shape (a typical example being an increase or decrease in weight depending on the time of year; exercise; any health issues that cause less movement) you must contact your saddle fitter. It is highly likely the saddle will no longer be fitting correctly and will either need some adjustment, or you may have to get a new saddle. If you notice any changes, for

What to Wear

example, if your saddle has started to move, get it checked as soon as you possibly can.

The bridle also needs to be the right size for your horse – it cannot be too small so that it is always pulling at their mouth or dragging on their ears and giving them a headache. What about those double reins and the martingale? Do you really need them? If you were able to understand better what your horse wants and is comfortable in, maybe you wouldn't have to fight them so much on every ride.

Tack that *looks* quality is a big thing for us – we all like matching sets and looking as well turned out as we can (I blame childhood gymkhanas for this!), but if it does not fit your horse comfortably and is causing them problems, then you might as well get used to having a horse that lunges for you every time you do up the girth. Having a fancy name and an enormous price tag does not necessarily mean that the tack is any good – well, it's probably good quality, but if it's no good for your horse, then it's no good for you either.

Some horses are very particular about their tack; most clients I have are trying to do the best for their horses, and as such they have piles of saddles, bridles, rugs, headcollars, boots – and everything else. But, if a horse likes a certain saddle for the comfort, you are better off listing the rest on eBay, because the horse will not be happy otherwise! One horse I communicated with told me, in no uncertain terms, that his owner should use a particular bridle that he had been unsure about using because it looked like something from *Star Trek*. However, it was the most comfortable for the horse and he knew what he needed to be able to do his job well.

Interestingly, a lot of us are getting into the idea of 'anatomical bridles', which are designed to remove some of the pressure on the poll. This is all well and good, but that pressure then has to go somewhere – whether that be on the nose or elsewhere on the face. I have noticed that anatomical bridles are generally not the favourite of horses. Obviously, I don't want to name brands or prices here, but I will say that I know of a popular anatomical bridle, which is nowhere near as good as other, lesser-known counterparts available on the market. It's just a case of trial and error, which I realise is not very helpful advice.

The thing is, we are all different and so are our horses. Your friend may be comfortable and beautiful in an outfit that would pinch you in all sorts of unspeakable places – and it's the same with our horses. One size definitely does not fit all. Some horses are fine in just a bog-standard headcollar; others need a little more pressure in certain places and so would be better off with one of the Parelli halters. Some are perfectly happy striding out in an old saddle that has been through many horses before; others are more 'princess and the pea' types who need their tack made to measure.

The key is to make sure that the tack you are using is fitted correctly to your horse. Their shape and size fluctuate over the course of the year, depending on what they eat and how much exercise they are getting. Just because a piece of tack fitted your horse perfectly last year, does not mean it will still fit perfectly this year.

Different tack is designed for different purposes. You wouldn't go on a six-hour trail ride in a jumping saddle, would you? (Pro tip – you should definitely not do this.) The tack needs to be suitable for the job the horse is doing.

Another thing to consider is your position on the horse. If you are sitting heavier on one side than another, this will affect the wear of the saddle on one side or the other. Using a mirror when schooling, or getting a friend to walk behind you on a ride to check your position will help you to figure out what your body does when you ride.

Noseband fitting is another big thing – I hear from a lot of horses that the noseband is constricting their nasal passages, because it is not fitting or sitting in the right way. Get it checked out! Make sure it fits well – no one can work efficiently if they can't breathe.

Browbands are another issue – horses also get headaches. Pressure from a hat that is too tight is very uncomfortable, isn't it? Next time you're out and about, spare a thought for your horse's browband and make sure that it is comfortable for them. You should be able to comfortably run a finger underneath it, while having it fit snugly around the poll.

Bitting can be another sticky issue. The bit must be correctly fitted and it must be suited for the job the horse is doing. You really don't need a Pelham on that happy hacker while you are plodding around the lanes. Yes, we all like brakes and the ability to not be tanked off with. But you want the horse to be listening to your seat and voice, and not having to be hanging off their mouths wherever you can possibly avoid it.

Bitless bridles work really well for some horses, and there are more and more options out there for this type of bridle, which is even permitted in showjumping and eventing these days. These are two of the most dangerous sports, so this is a great recommendation for the efficacy of this method. As I say, you know your own horse and how sensitive they are to brakes and steering. Pick whatever works for you and them, while keeping you both safe and comfortable. Bitless bridles work for some horses, not for others. I'm not going to get into the ins and outs of this one because everyone has their own opinion – if it works for you, fine. If it doesn't, fine. The principle is still the same though – the bridle must fit well, and you must avoid hanging off the reins.

While we're on the reins and bit subject, I do recommend getting a neckstrap. These are great because if your horse suddenly spooks or shies, you have something to grab hold of that is not the softest part of your horse's anatomy – their mouth. Sometimes, as we all know, there is nothing you can do but hang on – and in this situation, you don't want to be hanging on to their mouths. I always tell people that if a neckstrap is good enough for William Fox-Pitt, then it's good enough for the rest of us!

Rugs can also be a bit of a sore subject. When to rug? How often? What weight? Should you change your horse's rug because everyone else at the yard has switched to heavyweight, and you wonder if you are doing the right thing? Should you even rug at all?

This question, like so many others, is based on personal preference – yours and your horse's. If you have a shaggy native, you may find that they can get through the year without any extra coverings at all. Your thin-skinned Arab may start shivering and dropping weight at the first sign of the leaves turning – they are all different.

As with the tack, the most important thing to do is to ensure that your rugs fit correctly. The chances are your horse will be wearing it for hours or days at a time, so make certain that there are no rubbing places, no patches where it can cause damage to the coat or the skin underneath, and that all the straps sit comfortably and are not twisted. Just imagine going out in your nice warm winter coat and finding that it rubs and chafes in uncomfortable places – not a nice thought, is it?

Once you have found the right clothing for you and your horse, I can promise you that many of the issues that can come with poorly fitting tack – nasty faces; bucking and bronking; napping; rearing and even a plain old refusal to work – will disappear, almost overnight. Instead of a bag of carrots, get your horse the gift of a really thorough saddle fitting for Christmas this year.

10

OILS

Occasionally, I will pick up from a horse that they are deficient in something in their diet, or that they would benefit from some added extras to improve their health, both mental and physical. Essential oils are a part of these added extras, and I will often encourage clients to use a certain essential oil to help their horse to think, to focus, or to simply relax.

Essential oils are made directly from the plant, generally using a distillation method. The plant that is useful is extracted, compressed, concentrated, so that you end up with an oil that is the exact smell of the plant it came from – with all the properties of the plant contained within it. It may sound strange to think that a smell can help our horses, but when you think of the olfactory abilities of a horse, compared to our own, and how you might become slightly more relaxed or invigorated around certain smells, it makes sense.

When applied to the skin, essential oils can pass right into the bloodstream through the dermal layers, where they can get to work on whatever they need to do. Even when they are not applied directly to the skin, oils will set about doing their work. The smell of the oils reaches the emotional centre of the brain – if we are using these things to help our horses *feel* a certain way, this is exactly what we want them to do. Horses are incredibly sensitive to smells – they

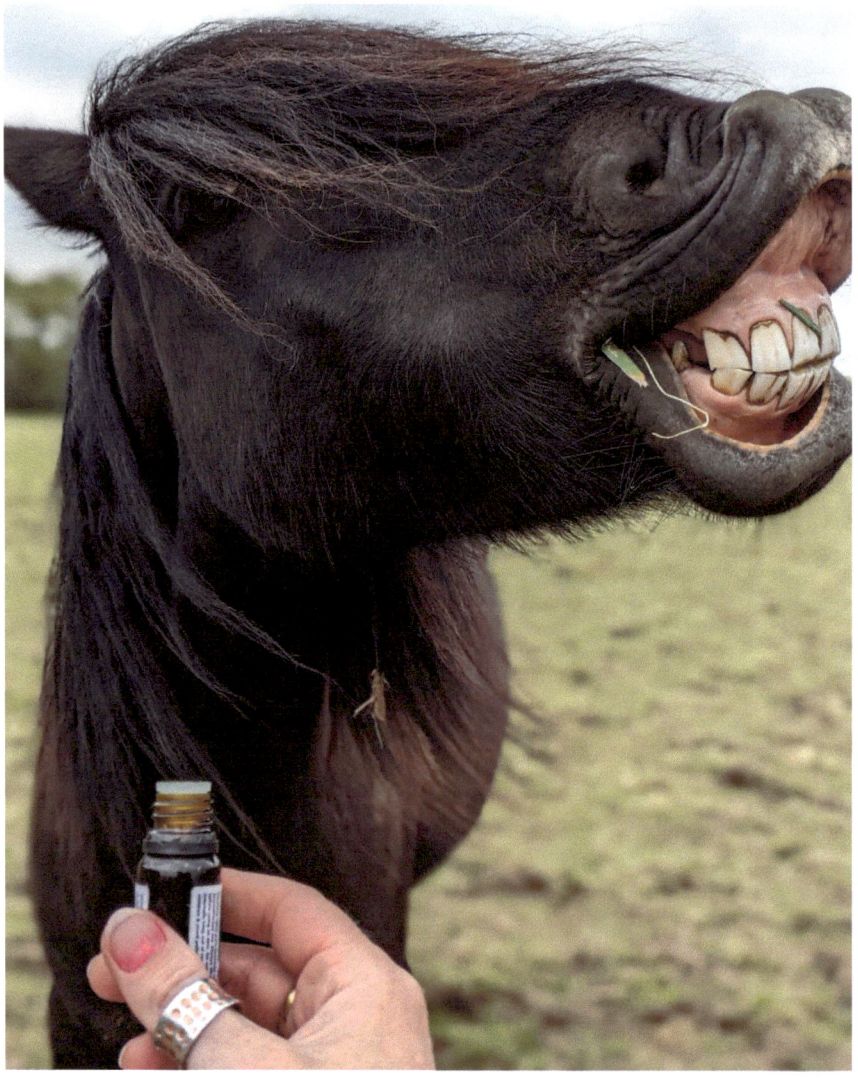

Some horses react quite startlingly to essential oils! (Faith Hancock)

use their olfactory senses to work out what foods are good; to bond mother and foal; to detect the presence of predators, and to work out where they are. This is partly why they are so open to the use of oils in everyday life – smelling things is a big part of their lives.

There is a whole branch of essential oils used for animals that is called zoopharmacognosy – this is where you present the horse with a variety of different essential oils and they will be immediately drawn to one or two of them, and when you look into the properties of these two oils, it turns out that they are eminently suitable for your horse and their particular issues. There are people out there who do this for a living, and I don't want to tread on any toes, so I don't make this the biggest part of my job. However, I do know that some horses can benefit enormously from oils, so I will recommend them where I see fit and whether or not the client decides to follow my recommendations is up to them.

Horses are very sensitive, and they do not have the mental blocks that some people might have regarding aromatherapy. Interestingly, they instinctively sniff the oils in just the way that they are most effective. They first sniff with one nostril which connects to one side of the brain, then with the opposite one, which links into the other side of the brain. If the oil is not beneficial to them, they will turn away and show no interest, but if you hit on the right oil, they will be much more engaged.

Most essential oils are also fine for horses to lick at, and some of them will do so very enthusiastically, if you get the right oil – but I would not recommend allowing them to lick at oregano, tea tree or any of the other 'hot' oils. This is the fastest way to turn your horse off essential oils; if you've ever accidentally got oregano oil in your mouth then you will understand why! None of these oils are poisonous or dangerous to your horses, it's just that some of them are extremely unpalatable.

Essential oils can have a dramatic effect on horses. You can watch a snorting, plunging, crazy pile of flying hooves and snaking necks turn into a docile donkey after a sniff or two of the right oil. A horse that turns itself inside out when its herd mate leaves the field can suddenly relax and start grazing, with the correct application of the right oil.

Using oils can be a tricky business – there are so many of them out there and it can be really hard to know where to start.

There are a good few that I always keep in my tack box, and that I recommend to clients because I know they work, without fail, for some of the more common issues such as hot-headedness, separation anxiety, and difficulties concentrating.

Some oils will have a dramatic effect when horses simply sniff them, others can be applied topically. You can apply antifungal and antimicrobial oils on to wounds and to help deal with foot issues – just be careful and make sure you dilute them with a carrier oil if you are applying to wound sites, so that they don't burn the skin– while others, such as lavender, can be freely applied to the whole of your horse to help them deal with stressful conditions.

I normally recommend a topical application – when it is not a wound that is being dealt with – that focuses on the ears, the poll and the top of the head. The oils can be absorbed by the skin and their effects will usually be immediately apparent – sometimes incredibly dramatically. Don't worry if your horse is not up for having oils spread all over his head – sniffing the oils and even licking them will have just the same effect.

I am not an aromatherapist, but I do know about essential oils – I know that they work and what effect certain oils will have on a particular type of horse. I have a few oils that I consistently suggest that owners use on their horses, because having a calm horse who has been able to quieten their mind has got to be a good thing.

Lavender

This one is well known for its calming, relaxing properties – in fact, it's in just about every bath product for babies on the market today. Lavender will help to relax the body and the mind – something that is ideal when we are working with horses. It has the same effect on the calmest of horses to the most volcanic. It is pretty impressive to watch a horse chill out completely once they sniff at a phial of lavender.

Sweet orange
This is another calming oil; it's great for horses who are a bit wild, or those that are easily stressed. It's simultaneously a mood uplifter and a calmer – I know these things don't always go together, but there we are. It's well worth trying if you have either a horse that needs cheering up, or one that needs calming down. Surprisingly, it will work wonders on either type. This oil is also a boost for the immune system and it can help to reduce the spread of airborne bacteria, which is great for your horse if you are liveried at a yard and respiratory problems are going round.

Blue yarrow
This one is a very good all-round oil, with particular focus on anti-inflammation. Inflammation is a cause of many problems with horses (and people), so reducing an inflammation can lead to a whole bunch of different – and more agreeable – behaviours. Yarrow is great for respiratory issues and is a good one to turn to if your horse suffers from seasonal allergies. A sniff of yarrow on the days that the pollen count is sky-high can work wonders.

Rosemary
You may have heard about this oil as a memory stimulant, used by students studying for exams, and as such it's great for older horses and those who might seem to be a bit forgetful. It can also help to stimulate the appetite and I have used it successfully with a horse that was anorexic (yes, horses can share our mental-health issues, too), and it can assist in reminding them to eat the things that are good for them.

Jasmine
This oil is very calming and one that is great for horses that are afraid and prone to spooking. It can also help to calm a headstrong, bargy horse due to its stress-relieving properties. It is good for the

physical body, being used to reduce inflammation, ease muscle pain and improve circulation of the body. Jasmine can also be used to lift the mood of horses who seem low and it is a great general energiser and spirit-lifter. This one is good for horses who feel separation anxiety when their friends are taken from the field.

Peppermint
You have probably heard about how peppermint is good for the digestion. Well, peppermint oil is very good for horses that are struggling with gut health issues. Simply breathing it in will benefit their bodies, and if they lick it then that's fine, too. It is also very helpful as a concentration aid, so will be ideal for those horses whose minds seem to wander away from the task at hand!

Grapefruit
This oil has twofold properties; it is associated with the liver and can be used to help break down fats more effectively. It is a great natural cleanser, for both people and horses, and smelling it is incredibly uplifting. It can help to raise the mood with those horses who seem low and sluggish.

Violet leaf
I love this one. It is brilliant for horses that are generally nervous and unsettled, and who tend to spook easily at little things. It's a great oil to give to a new horse who has just arrived on your yard and seems a little up in the air and unable to relax. It's also a good one for those who have moved homes many times and are showing signs of nervous exhaustion. It is said to comfort and strengthen the heart, so it's great to use for horses who have separation anxiety also.

Oregano
This is something that we should all keep in our tack boxes – oregano is one of the best antibacterial, antifungal and antimicrobial oils

that there is. You can use this one more topically than the others; it's great for abscesses and wounds that need to be cleaned. (Think of it as a purple spray without any other added ingredients.) However, oregano is a 'hot' oil that *should not* be applied directly to the skin without being diluted in a carrier oil first. This oil can be used neat on the feet for infection, thrush or seedy toe, but it *cannot* be used neat on any soft tissue, as it can burn and cause blistering.

Tea tree

An oil that we will probably all have heard of is tea tree, which is another great disinfectant and one that also should be used topically. It is very good mixed with salt water for wound bathing, and although it is not as strongly antifungal as oregano, it is a great antimicrobial and disinfectant. Tea tree can be applied directly to the skin, but you should dilute it for horses, especially if they have not had it applied before or are particularly sensitive.

If you want to look more into this subject then I encourage you to do so – aromatherapy is a wonderful thing, and it is often more noticeable in the effects it has on an animal, in the same way that it has with children. Often, those that do not have a set mind frame of 'Oh, this is weird and my doctor hasn't prescribed it to me, therefore I won't trust it!' will respond better to alternative therapies. Their minds are open, and they do not have any fixed areas of thinking that prevent them from accepting a different form of treatment, just because it's different.

Essential oils can help improve so many things about your horse's behaviour by doing nothing more than buying a few of the oils and letting them have a sniff! If you are interested, there are numerous books available that can enable you to learn more about the subject and how it can help.

I would suggest learning as much as you can about the different plants that are used, because often the applications in plant form are different from using them as essential oils. You can experiment with a few different oils and see which ones your horse decides to go for – the results may well surprise you. There are so many out there and it is really easy to get hold of them – just make sure, as I always advise with any supplement, that you get the most natural, preferably organic and non-GMO versions that you possibly can.

One last point to make is that if you compete at a level where you have the possibility of being blood tested, it is definitely worth being mindful about the calming oils you use. These can sometimes cause problems with the blood tests, so it's probably best to avoid these in the week of any such competition.

11

CASE STUDIES

Over the years, I have worked with a large number of horses and clients. I've been doing this for a good while now, and countless horses and their owners have benefited from a bit of outside help. I wanted to include some of their stories, because to hear from the horse's mouth (sorry for the pun!) what they have said, and how communicating with them has improved their lives and those of their owners, is very important. Many thanks to everyone who has contributed – these people, have written their stories in their own words, for which I am very grateful.

I find it very interesting to note how many of my clients have started out incredibly cynical about what I do, but they had literally nowhere else to turn. After I worked with them, they were suddenly able to better understand their horses and improve not only their physical health but also many different types of behavioural issues.

Without these real-life stories from clients, I could appear to be one of those dubious people, putting up smokescreens to make you believe that I am some kind of magical guru. I'm not. I just care about your horses. I hope you enjoy reading these accounts as much as I have enjoyed working with the horses and their people.

Dulcibella – Faith Hancock

I am Cheryl's author and my story is not as wild as some, but having discovered Cheryl I feel her gift needs to be shared – hence this book. I hope you don't mind my slipping in the story of my horse before anyone else's.

I first found out about Cheryl through a friend of mine who was having her horse read. I managed to book an appointment for Dulcibella, my eighteen-month-old Warlander. I bought Dulcie in 2022, having lost my own beloved homebred heart horse, Venus, to horrendous colic two years previously. There was a hole in my life that couldn't be filled by anything else; I wasn't replacing Venus, but I needed another horse to love.

I fell in love with Dulcie's cheeky little confident self and brought her home several months after she was weaned. She was so confident and so people-oriented that it was hard to find any boundaries! She would chase us around in the field, legs waving, trying to 'play'. Now I'm all for liberty training, but I draw the line at back hooves flying around inches from my face, when they're attached to a very pushy youngster who is going to grow to the size of a mountain. Dulcie had also taken against my mum, who has three other horses in the same field, and used to lunge out and bite her. One particularly nasty bite to the face made me seriously think I should find a different home for this girl. This, along with the fact that the rest of the horses appeared to hate her and were very aggressive towards her, made our herd very uncomfortable.

Cheryl's reading made me feel so much more confident with this bright star, and having found out that she didn't like Mum because 'her head's always in the clouds', has made it so much easier for us all to get along. I was astonished that Cheryl knew my mum was an Aquarius, simply based on what Dulcie, a Taurus with Aries tendencies, had said about

Case Studies

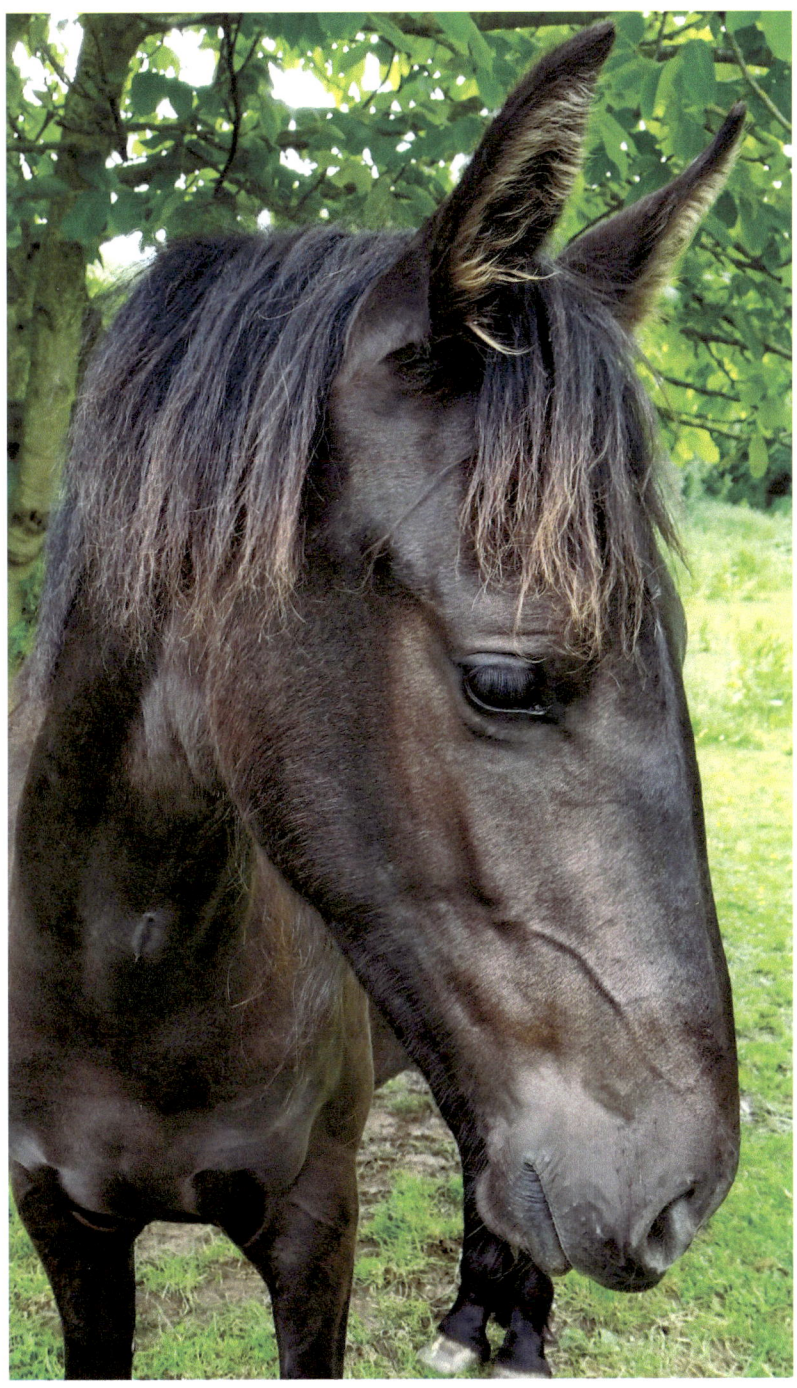

Dulcibella. (Faith Hancock)

her frustrations with not being concentrated on properly. I was given recommendations for essential oils to help calm her, and it's astonishing to see how she responds to this. Cheryl was able to pick up on the adjustments to Dulcie's back that my McTimoney chiropractor had done the week before, and described our pasture perfectly from doing a body scan and noticing how healthy her liver was.

During Dulcie's reading, Cheryl also picked up on a 'strong, maternal feeling' in the field. Obviously this wasn't Dulcie, she was too young for babies – so we moved on to Flo, the mother of my previous girl (Venus). I quickly sent over a picture of Flo's eye and, out of nowhere, Cheryl told me, 'This horse is heartbroken.' Of course, I burst into floods of tears, the loss of Venus being still so painful. I hadn't told Cheryl about Venus previously, as we were there to discuss Dulcie. However, Cheryl knew, from the feeling of the field and from looking into Flo's eye, exactly what was going on.

Since then, we have all spent a lot of time telling Flo that we loved Venus, that she will never be forgotten, that Flo was a wonderful mum, and that of course it wasn't her fault. I also tell her that Dulcie is *not* a replacement for her beloved daughter, and now Dulcie and Flo are often grazing together. The aggression has completely vanished.

The entire vibe of the herd has changed – Dulcie is no longer aggressive, Flo is her usual stoic self, and everything is calm and peaceful. It is incredible how much can change just by understanding the horses better. Thank you, Cheryl.

Spanish – Tayah Birkett

Spanish is a seventeen-year-old Pura Raza Espanol, who I bought on a whim as a rescue from Spain. She'd had a terrible start in life and wasn't expected to survive. Because

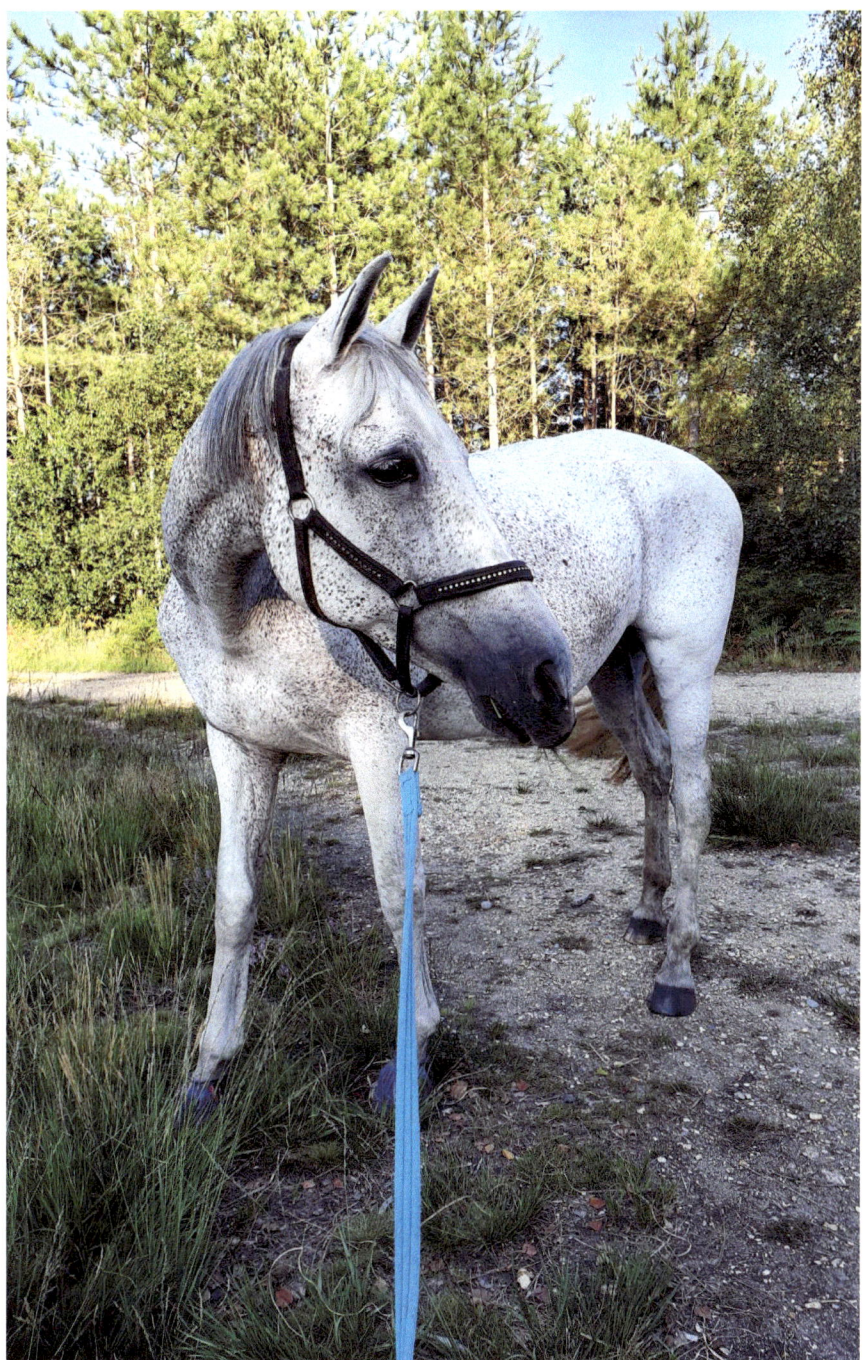

Spanish. (Tayah Birkett)

of this, she had severe trust issues, was a nightmare to ride and even to handle. She would rear up under saddle and go over backwards, and was generally very difficult to be around. She had undergone scans for absolutely everything, including MRI scans to rule out anything physical that was causing the behavioural problems. She was given a completely clean bill of health by the vet, and we were at a loss.

Cheryl was treating other horses at the same yard, and when she started to talk to Spanish everything became much clearer. Because of her troubled past, she had huge issues about food, and we discovered that she was always hungry and afraid that she'd be left without food. Spanish also told Cheryl that she felt bad for her ridden behaviour, but that her saddle was really hurting her and she just couldn't help trying to stop the pain.

Once we had fixed these issues, Cheryl helped us get to the point that we could hack Spanish out sensibly (well, nine times out of ten anyway!) and she was even placed in a dressage competition. We thought we were in the clear.

Then, out of the blue, poor Spanish was diagnosed with liver disease and given eight weeks to live. We were told to say our goodbyes as she could suddenly deteriorate and need to be euthanised any day. I asked Cheryl to come back again, so that Spanish could tell us how she was feeling and to see if there was anything else we could do. Cheryl helped us to realise that not giving up is very important, and how a mindset can change issues in the physical body. She also advised us to start on high doses of milk thistle and had her 'psychic surgeon' friend join us for a few sessions.

After a few weeks, we had Spanish's blood retested and all came back clear. She was tested weekly for several months, with the same results, and on Christmas Eve my vet phoned to say, 'We cannot explain this scientifically, but Spanish is completely recovered.'

Spanish is now retired and is much more relaxed than she was – all my staff can now catch her, and she stands calmly to allow her blood to be taken for testing every few months. She is a complete poppet, and I am so very thankful for having had the opportunity to work with Cheryl, who I genuinely believe has saved this horse's life.

Arizona Pie – Louise McPherson

I bought Pie from a dealer in May 2018; she is now nineteen and is a 15.2hh Appaloosa. I didn't know anything about Pie's history and I really wanted to find out more about her past, so I found Cheryl on Facebook. I was overwhelmed by her insight – she got Pie's personality spot-on, even though she had never met her. She told me that Pie had been passed from pillar to post, and sometimes mistreated (this was clear from Pie's difficult and sometimes aggressive behaviour).

Pie then moved to my friend's place for a few months, to be company for my friend's horse who had recently lost his companion. Well, Pie decided she didn't want to be there, and escaped and found her way back home! It soon became clear that she wasn't well, and Cheryl told me that it 'felt' like sycamore poisoning. There was indeed a sycamore at my friend's place and, yes, Pie had become sick from it. The vet came and told me that all we could do was hope for the best overnight. In a panic, I called Cheryl. She was out shopping at the time but stopped everything to perform some long-distance reiki healing on Pie. Thankfully, she pulled through, and I do credit Cheryl with this recovery.

Since then, we have had more sessions with Cheryl – including a reading for a loan horse, Minnie, when Pie was feeling lazy and didn't want to talk! Again, Minnie's reading was spot-on, and I feel that we all communicate better silently since we have had Cheryl involved.

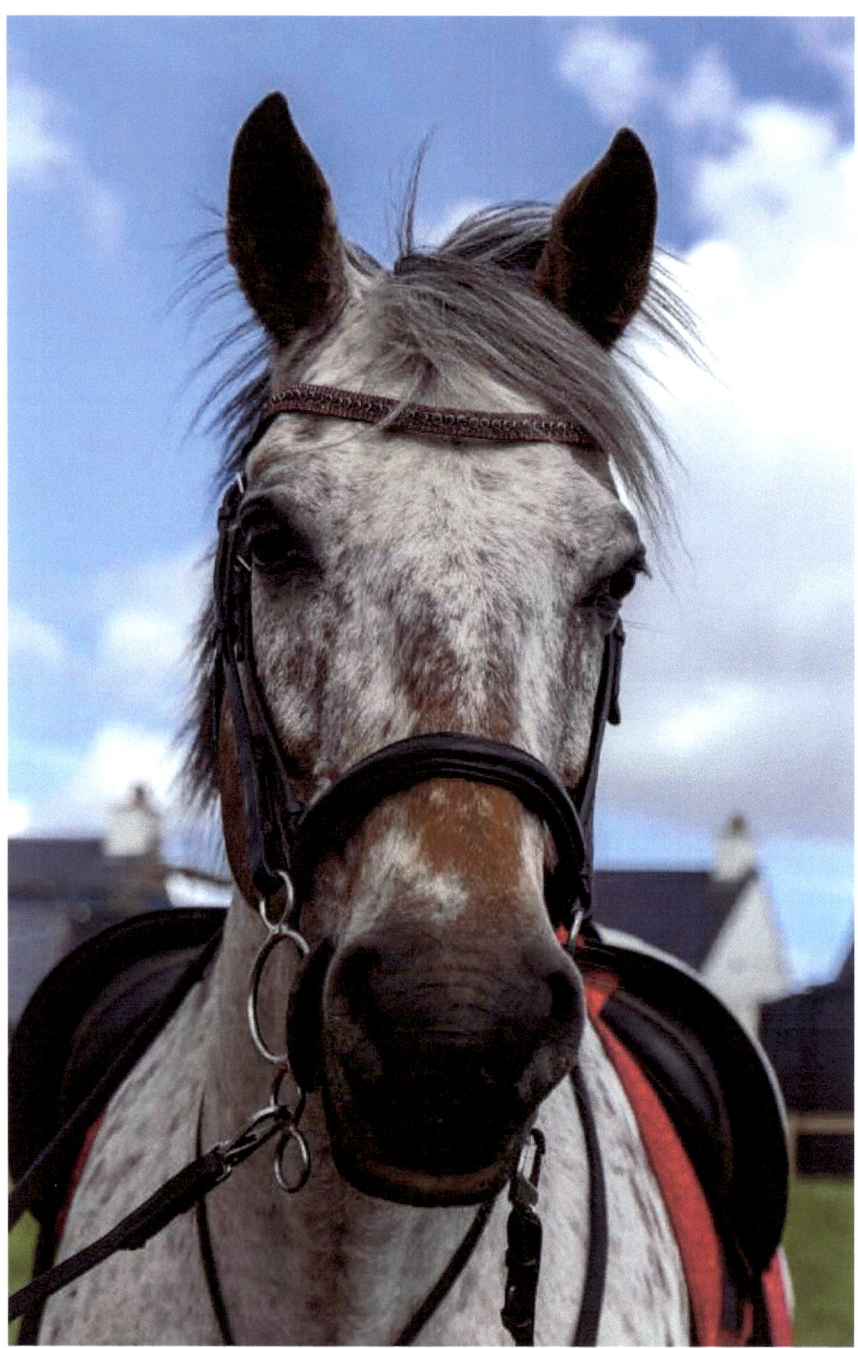

Arizona Pie. (Louise McPherson)

Case Studies

George and Lorcan – Jane Sandever

George is a seventeen-year-old New Forest, standing at 13.2hh. We'd had George for some time, when he suddenly started being nasty and aggressive. He would charge at people in the field, try to bite and kick, and it was only me who was allowed to go anywhere near him – and he would sometimes not even tolerate me. When we found Cheryl, she came out to see George who was in the stable at the time, pacing around and looking very unhappy and aggressive. The first thing he said to Cheryl was, 'I hurt people. I don't mean to.'

We found out through Cheryl that our boy had been separated from his mum when he was too young and placed in a stable with both doors shut, so he felt alone, scared and heartbroken. We since found out that this was standard treatment for the 'spirited' ones.

Once we found out what George had been through, we took the time to understand him and treat him with gentle loving kindness, and our bond has improved over the years. George is an absolute legend, and he will be with us forever.

Lorcan, our 15.2hh Irish sports horse, was bought for my daughter as a competition horse. As he settled in, his personality seemed to change – because of our experiences with George, we called out Cheryl straight away. She told us that Lorcan would improve, but that he was suffering from a breakdown – he certainly was a horse who displayed a lot of anxiety traits. We were advised to turn him out 24/7 so he would get the benefit of a natural, stress-free life – in fact, Cheryl told us he was literally screaming out for this.

When Cheryl came back again, Lorcan was a different horse. His floodgates opened and he told us that the dealer had worked him ferociously hard, and that even a blood test wouldn't show what he had been given to sedate him before he came to us.

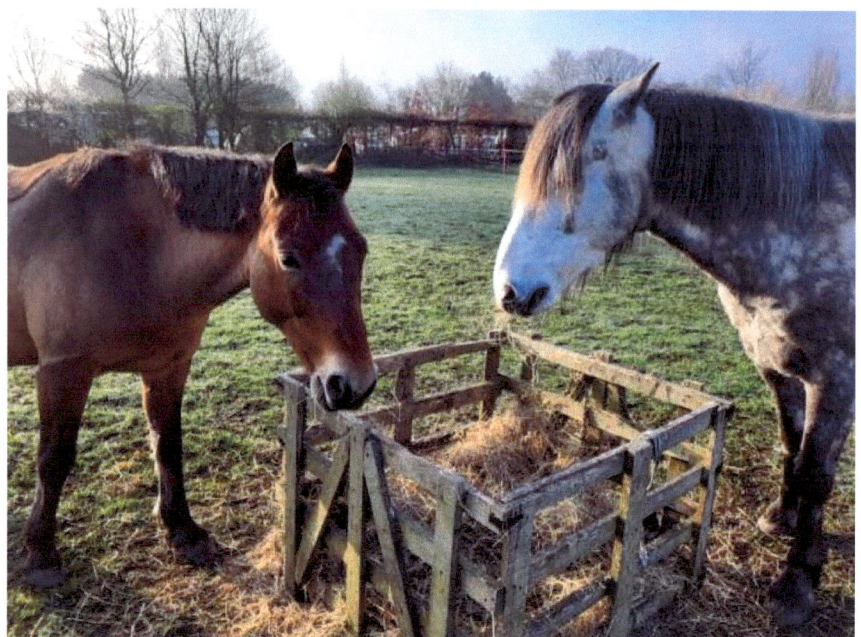

George and Lorcan. (Jane Sandever)

With the time off in the field, he started to realise that he could trust us and that we only wanted the best for him. He is now an absolute pleasure to work with, and he and George also have a fantastic relationship. By taking the time to listen, Cheryl helped both our boys to tell us what was going on with them, so that we could help to improve their lives, and I will be forever grateful.

'Henry' – Lynne Perry

Henry (not his real name, and there's no photo of this horse because he wants to maintain his privacy) is a high-level dressage horse, a homebred warmblood standing at 16.1hh. I wanted help with Henry, as he was very reluctant to bend to the right – obviously an essential skill for a dressage horse! Initially, Cheryl identified some pain in the right ribcage and also a restriction in him breathing deeply. Cheryl suggested contacting a Bowen practitioner, which I did, and I definitely noticed some improvement.

Next, we started working with the Bowen practitioner and Cheryl both present while I was riding; Cheryl would identify a problem area, the Bowen practitioner would address it, then I would get back on to see if there was an improvement. There was an improvement, every single time.

Henry is now working really well, and because he is a horse with so much top-level potential, I am so pleased to have found Cheryl to help us work through his issues. As well as his physical problems, Cheryl was spot-on with his personality, which in turn has helped us to work together better and be even more in tune than before.

Dev – Hannah Tomo

I bred Dev, whose full name is Endeavour, and was there at her birth – she's now ten and is a part-bred Arab of 14.3hh (though she's pretty sure she's much bigger than this!). Dev was the perfect pony until she was around six – this was when my sweet little friend turned into a bit of a devil. She went from happily giving and receiving cuddles, to a wild creature who would lunge at me with her teeth bared. I was wary about seeking veterinary advice, as I'd previously had bad experience with my practice, so I bit the bullet and called Cheryl.

I should tell you that I am the *biggest* cynic and didn't think for one minute that Cheryl would be able to tell me anything about my horse that I didn't already know. I was very guarded with the information I gave her and only shared the briefest of details. I was floored with the reading that came back – Cheryl 'knew' things that she had no chance of knowing unless my horse was truly communicating with her.

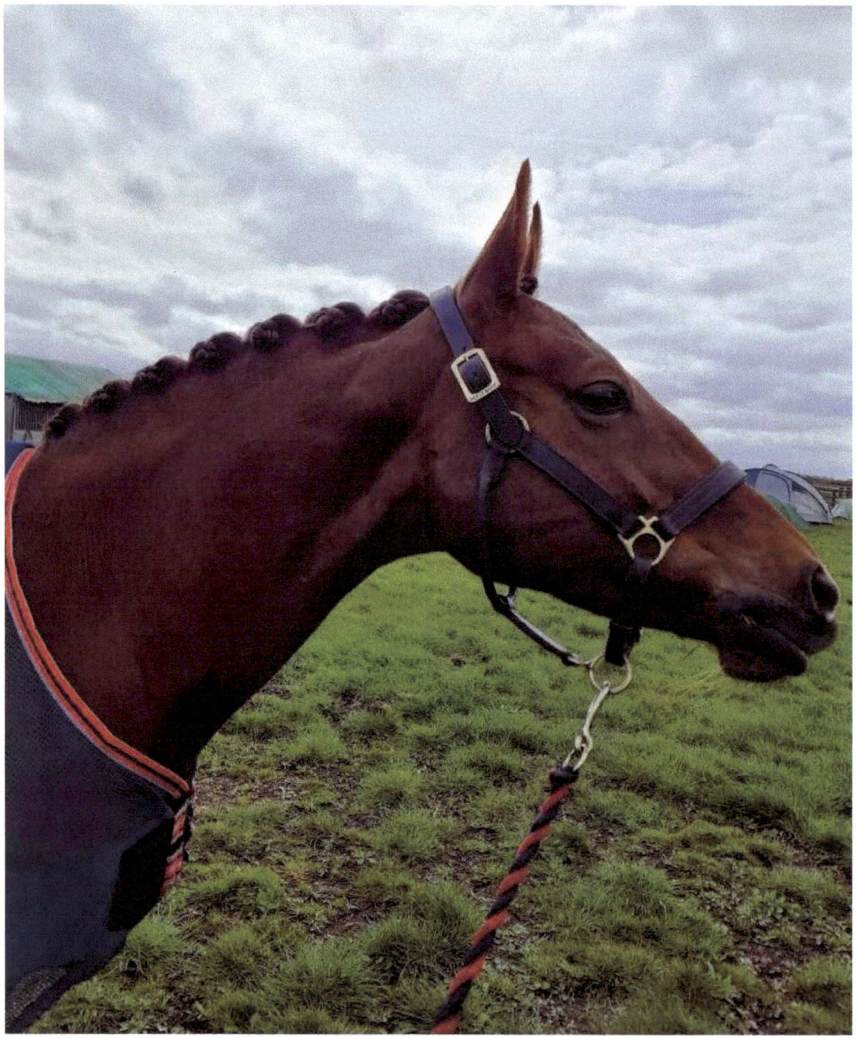

Dev. (Hannah Tomo)

Now, Dev is a chestnut mare and, as such, a lot of people simply put her behaviour down to being 'just a chestnut mare', but I was blown away when Cheryl told me how much pain she was in. Cheryl said it was her *near-side* shoulder, and it was recommended that we seek Bowen therapy for her. The treatment started out quietly enough, but as Marion, the Bowen therapist, got round to Dev's near-side shoulder, Dev went through the roof. I started shouting at Marion to get out of the stable – I was genuinely worried that Dev was going to kill her!

However, she pushed through, got the release, and everything suddenly relaxed. Marion then rested her head on Dev's shoulder, started to laugh and told us, 'I've been trying to catch that girl out for years.' Marion had spotted that the *off-side* pecs were twitching as Dev trotted up and was sure that Cheryl was wrong in saying it was the near-side, but as it turned out, she was spot-on.

There were other, smaller things I learned that day, too, apparently my lorry made Dev feel seasick. I checked the tyre pressures, and lo and behold it was all out on one side. Dev told Cheryl about the different saddles we had tried, and the places in her body where she felt pain, and with this knowledge we were able to successfully treat her. Once all the places Cheryl had identified were treated, my sleepy-eyed, relaxed, loving little pony came back to me; she's still a chestnut mare, but she no longer lives up to the stereotype.

It was nothing short of miraculous – and as I said, I am incredibly cynical about this sort of thing. I am very happy to be eating my words now – and so is Dev.

Brandy and Sugarfoot – Emmy Doherty

Brandy is an Irish sports horse, standing at 15.2hh and she is fifteen years old. I bought her in 2021 and I just wanted to know a bit about her past before I had her. She was very aggressive around food and previously she had been called 'dangerous'. I wanted to find out what had happened to her, if she was happy to have babies, what discipline she liked to be ridden in – and anything else she might have wanted me to know.

I asked if Brandy wanted a foal; the answer was a very strong positive and she was insistent that she'd have a colt.

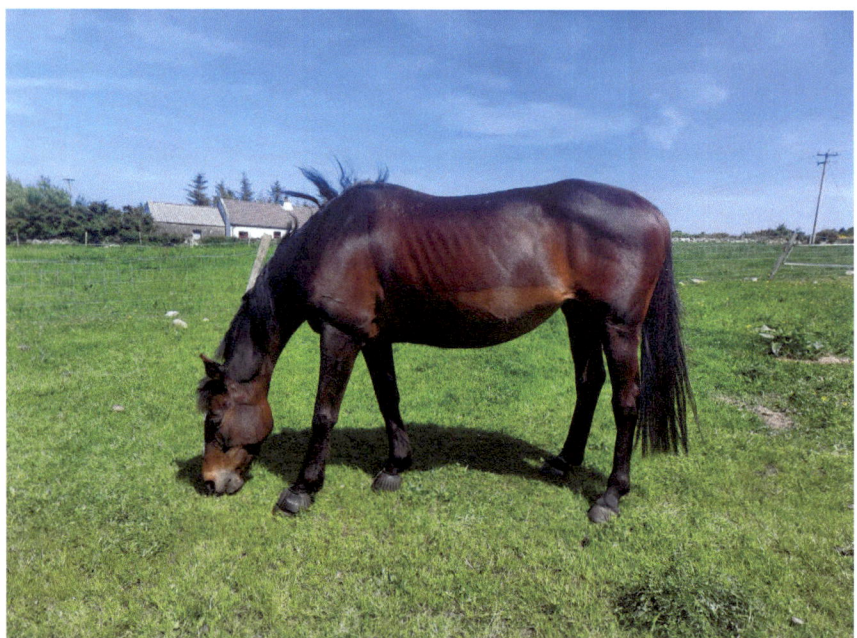

Brandy. (Emmy Doherty)

I was told about her feed issues – Brandy had said that she appreciated her food, but Cheryl told me that a certain type of horse food could cause her stomach issues, so that was dropped straight away.

Well, Cheryl answered 95 per cent of my questions before I'd even had a chance to ask them! As Brandy was very happy to be a mum, I got Cheryl in for a second, emergency reading as Brandy was giving birth. I was told that Brandy did want my help during her foaling; she wanted to start standing up and finish lying down (which she did) and delivered, with my help, the most beautiful, big filly. When she was *in utero*, we were convinced she was a colt, and in all my years I have never met a more 'boyish' filly!

Brandy and I now have the best relationship. She's still quirky, but thanks to Cheryl's insights I now feel more confident with reading her myself – I think sometimes we just

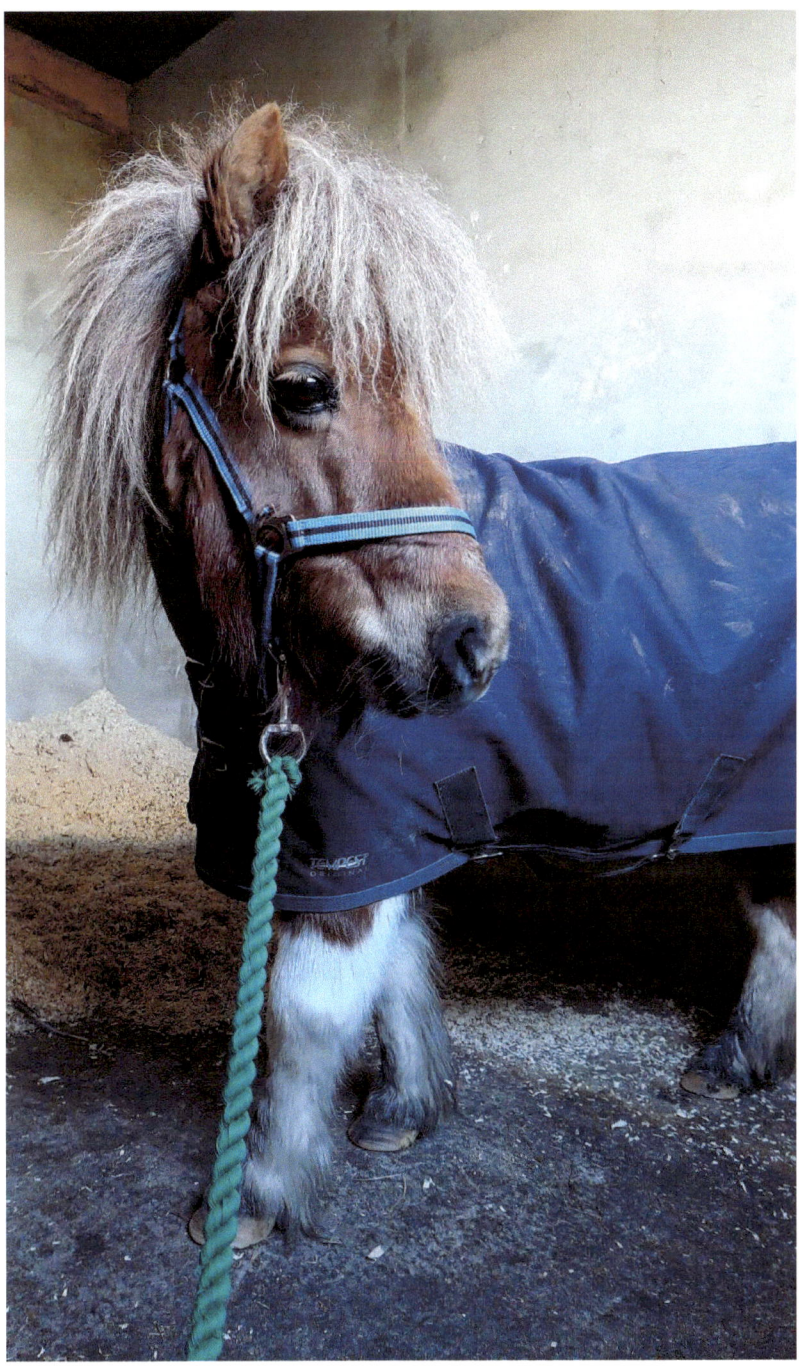

Sugarfoot. (Emmy Doherty)

need a little push to trust that voice in our heads, which is actually our horses talking to us.

Sugarfoot is a different story …

I bought her in 2021; she was ten when she arrived with us. She was always incredibly skittish and reluctant to come near us. I learned from Cheryl that Sugarfoot felt that she was far too good to be ridden; her job, she feels, is to keep everyone in place. She used the word 'dictator' to Cheryl, and this is pretty accurate! She is utterly fearless, despite her small size, and feels it is her job to protect us from anything. She is an escape artist (I can confirm this!) and she likes to be involved with everything. She looks in through the doors of the house and watches the dogs at the cooker – she thinks she'd fit in there quite well. Cheryl told us that she was 'Dolly Parton in horse form', and this fits so well with her personality.

It's so amazing to hear the things that I have thought about my horses, being voiced by my horses, through a lady who has never met them – and has no other vested interest in them. I know for a fact that Cheryl is the real deal.

Millie, Blackie, Missy and Midnight – Katie Coyle

I first learnt about Cheryl from a friend who was studying alongside me at a Therapeutic Riding Course in Wicklow. The first animal Cheryl read was my daughter's 14.2hh pony, who we were still trying to bond with even though we had owned her for a year. She can be a wee mare with attitude, which Cheryl picked up on and stated that she was an intelligent pony but can have a temper.

She described how Millie moved, and her ailments – which I had suspected and I was glad to have these confirmed. I had always noticed she had time for my son who has Down's syndrome, and I loved that Millie mentioned him to

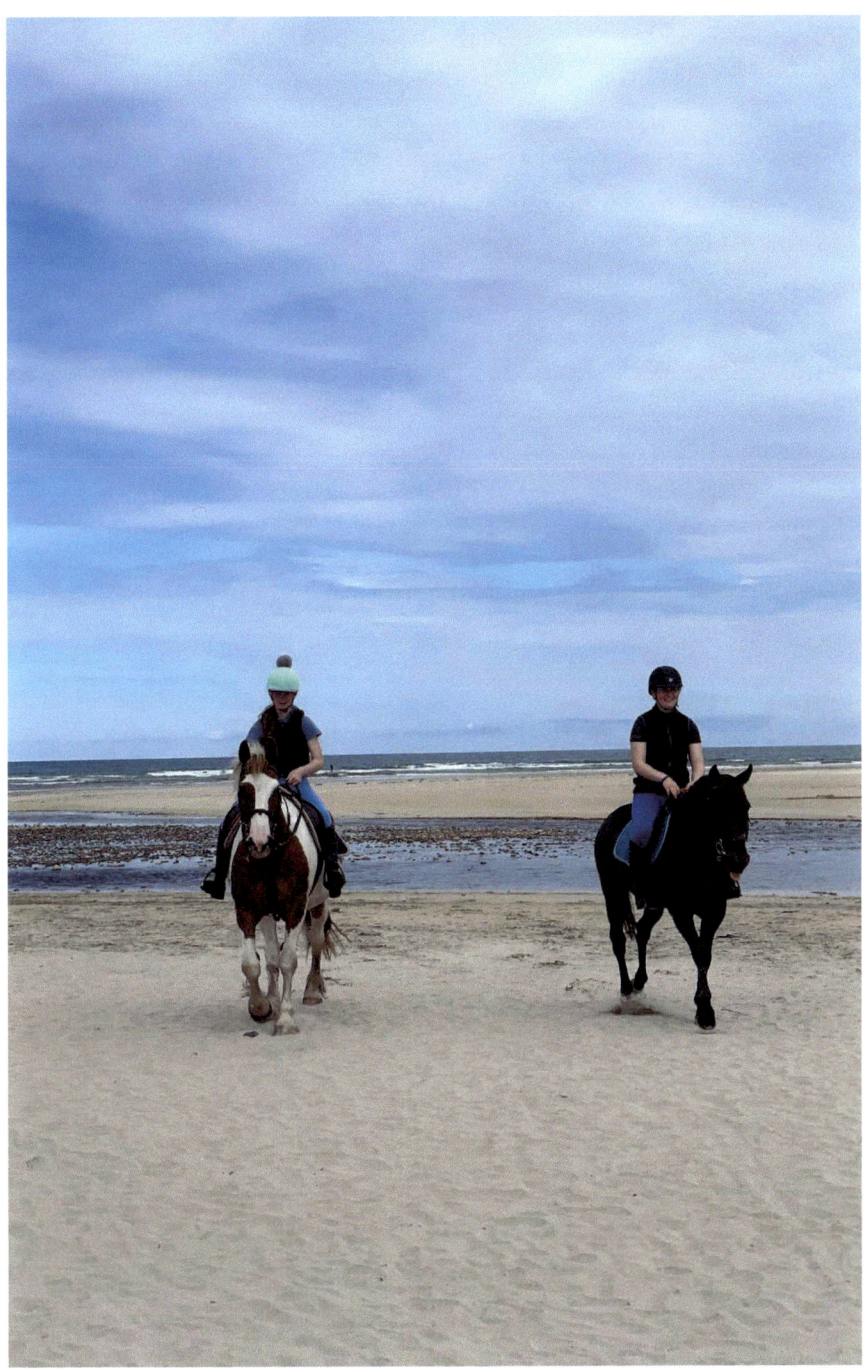

Millie and Missy. (Katie Coyle)

Cheryl and said that they had a special connection. Cheryl also advised us on top-to-toe health and dietary needs, which was of great use as so often we just chance our arm on a feed. We were even advised to arrange a Bowen treatment for Millie, which she loved and as I was the handler I feel I absorbed the healing properties, too.

So next I braved the insight of my thirty-three-year-old mare, Blackie, who I owned for twenty-eight years and who was always my confidante and rock, through good times and bad. Blackie's first statement was that she hated being called 'old' and that there was nothing wrong with her weight, so stop staring at her and worrying – she was just fine, thank you very much! Blackie stated that she had no patience for other horses, which I often noticed as she was 'a loner' in the field and was happy to be alone.

She adored me, was my best friend and sulked and stopped eating when I was away for a few days, which was confirmed by the rest of the family after the reading. Cheryl even described how she worked for me, her attitude and how she was always lively when ridden, although she never put us in danger.

She stated that 'it was a pleasure' when dealing with our son Joe – she was always so patient with him, but she was grumpy around other humans.

Again, we had a full body scan and feeding advice. This reading meant the most to me as this horse was my constant companion for so many years, and I was so relieved at the time that she was comfortable and healthy. Sadly, in February 2024, I had to have Blackie put down, but before making the decision I checked with Cheryl to see if she was ready to say goodbye. Thank God, Cheryl knew it was time.

Next was Missy, a horse I bought just after losing a wonderful pony who a vet tore while inseminating, and who we were going to try and get in foal with the frozen semen we had left after our tragic loss. Sadly, this didn't work but she was a perfect happy hacker or potential therapy horse.

Cheryl confirmed that Missy was a gentle horse who loved to be around people, was new to our yard, knew she wasn't being used much at the moment but was looking forward to working in a therapy setting, as she was a sensitive soul.

She described her previous owner to a tee, and it turned out that sadly he wasn't as kind to her as he appeared and could even be cruel to the point that she never felt good enough. Missy realises now that she is with us for life and really appreciates that.

Cheryl described how Missy can be awkward when pulling up the girth and getting the bit in, as she had been treated roughly before – but she is improving because we are gentle with her. Again, we were advised on feed for her and particular brands to avoid.

Missy had a bad accident when she managed to get barbed wire wrapped around her leg, an accident that Cheryl described despite not having been told about it – but noted that she had made a full recovery and may even be able to jump again, which she had always loved to do.

It was good to hear she was happy with us and loved that we were gentle with her, but it was so sad to hear she had been badly treated in her previous home, and even now I find it hard to see her previous owner when we are at shows where he is there.

I also got Cheryl to read two animals I have on our yard belonging to a friend which we use in the therapy business, too. First was Midnight who came from a riding school and seemed very closed off when she came, but after the reading, oh my goodness the difference in that wee pony! She now interacts with each rider, responds to their energy, licks and chews, relaxes when they have a release and regulate; it is truly magical.

Cheryl told us she had suffered huge trauma and we should constantly tell her we love her and that she is staying with us for life – and what a difference this has made in Midnight. She used to be difficult to catch, but now follows us around the field and just constantly interacts with us. Cheryl has brought us so much closer to all the animals, for which I will be forever grateful.

I have sent Cheryl's details to at least twenty people; they have all come back to me and thanked me as all the readings have been spot-on. She truly has the most amazing gift and I feel so lucky to have found her.

Dior and Zing – Susanne Allcroft

In the autumn of 2022, I felt that I was failing at life and particularly with my horses. During the spring I had lost my heart horse of twenty-three years who was the stalwart of the group, the confidence-giver and father figure and the steadying hand on the tiller. He left behind two mares who were not especially close. The atmosphere in the field had changed to one of lowness and isolation as the girls simply existed alongside one another but were not friends.

I decided to look for a companion horse so that I could carry on working with my young mare, Dior. In a strange twist of fate, following a national advert, Zing turned out to be just four miles away. He was a sad case; largely neglected, rescued from a horse hoarder, alone in a livery yard which was shortly to close down, and he refused to load onto a lorry or a trailer. So, I walked him home! After weeks of not being able to catch him, I found myself with two horses, both of whom were too worried to cope with anything more than life as a field ornament. Neither Dior nor Zing would leave the yard to hack out, and Dior became nervous and edgy in the manège.

I decided to send Cheryl a photograph of their eyes and have a reading. Luckily, I wrote notes and I often read them, amazed at what a fantastic insight they gave me into each horse's feelings and thoughts. I am convinced that Cheryl has helped me in this journey of understanding and working with both Dior and Zing, finding intense pleasure in spending time with them, and eventually starting to ride again, albeit taking small steps.

Dior's story

Cheryl told me 'Dior is very demanding and Zing allows her to get away with her behaviour' (now, he is always first to the gate but steps back to let her go first). 'She is suspicious and unforgiving of people who do her wrong, taking any affronts personally. She loves routine and can't cope with too many changes without having a meltdown. Although she is born under the sign of Taurus, she is much more Gemini in characteristics.'

I learnt from Cheryl to take small steps with her, to ensure that she understands what is happening, and to: 'Stop, rub her neck and bring her back into the room.' Giving Dior time to process information and reset has been hugely positive as Cheryl described her as 'slightly autistic'. With this in mind and knowing that eye contact and too much fuss can make her feel agitated, I now allow her to come to me on her terms. Having order, not cutting corners and seeing Dior last out of the three has worked well for her, and she is visibly more relaxed.

Dior has grown in confidence as predicted, she likes to 'eat, touch and push to understand' – I see this on a daily basis as she picks up, nudges and knocks over items

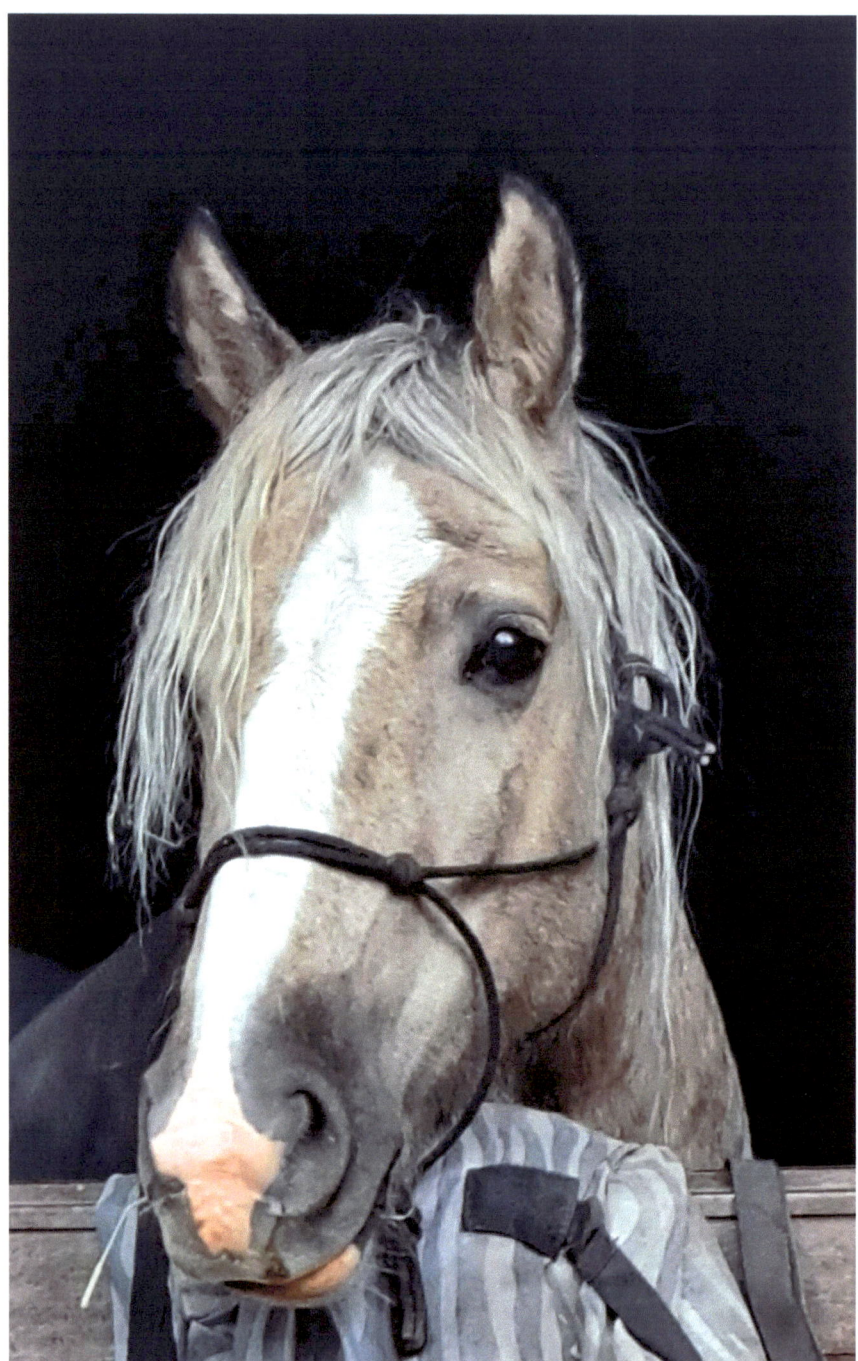

Dior. (Susanne Allcroft)

on the yard. She enjoys learning and loves the feeling of understanding the task, putting her head down when she feels comfortable.

Cheryl told me that Dior had some pain in her lower lumbar due to an accident on her near-side hind leg. I found this incredible as she badly cut her tendon on the near-side hind as a youngster and had her leg in plaster for ten weeks – Cheryl had no way of knowing this, and I hadn't told her. She suggested Bowen and I found a Bowen specialist who also worked holistically with Dior.

Although Dior has a 'can do' attitude in many ways, she lacks the confidence to lead on a hack and prefers to be side by side. She is sensitive and holds on to stuff; she looks stoic but is not. This helped me to understand her fears as it is easy to assume she is brave when she feels anxious. Lavender oil with aloe vera, and Bach's Rescue Remedy help her to feel less apprehensive.

Cheryl told me that Dior is pleased that I changed to a different farrier – I have an excellent farrier now, and Dior is barefoot. Her feet are much stronger and healthier than before. Knowing that she is happy in her daily life and is pleased that I took her on despite it being an inopportune time in my life, makes me happy every day – although I need to remind myself that my 'can do' energy is not always compatible with her introvert personality. She is complicated and marches to the beat of her own drum.

I asked why Dior suddenly stopped at a particular point on the drive and refused to go further. Cheryl told me that Prince (my old horse) had been going with her in spirit before but had now decided she could do it alone. Although this was heartbreaking to hear, it helped me to provide reassurance and comfort to her and I now feel we have an incredibly strong bond and understanding.

Zing's story

When Zing arrived, he had low self-esteem and felt that he was not interesting to ride or work with. He now understands his value and no longer feels like a second-class citizen! Zing is an all-round nice chap. He is gentle and takes a while to feel comfortable as he is often unsure, although he is not neurotic as some people describe him. He is super bright and enjoys consistency. My sign of Aries is very compatible with Zing, and I give him confidence, he loves me to talk to him. I often see this now as he stands in the field with me when I talk to him, and he closes his eyes.

Zing is sometimes 'there in body but not in mind', as he has coped in life by shutting down. He follows my body language, and now we do join-up successfully. Zing has brought out enthusiasm in my instructor that was waning for Dior; she enjoys working with him as he is receptive and bright when learning.

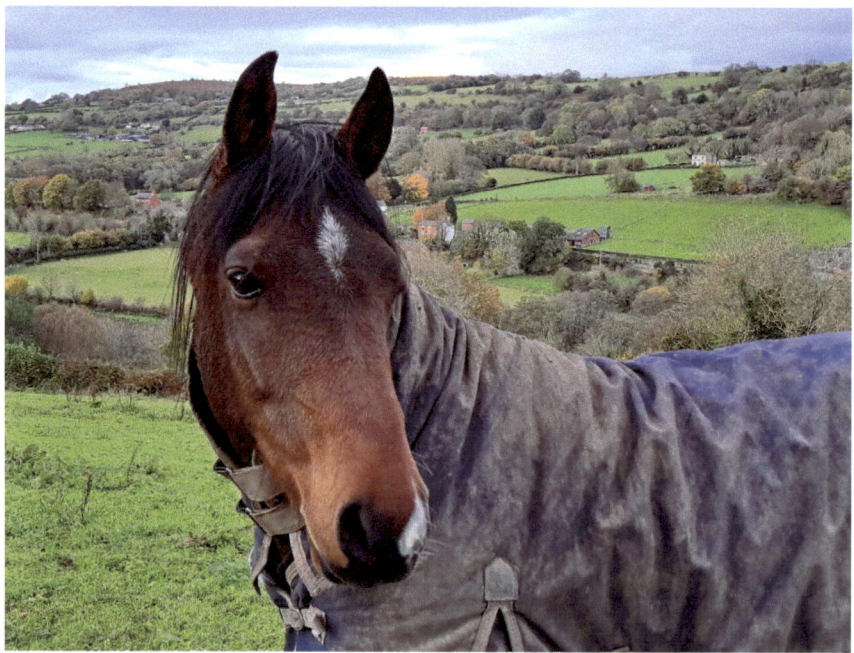

Zing. (Susanne Allcroft)

I didn't know much about Zing's history when Cheryl spoke to me. She told me that he hadn't been bitted and should be guided by my legs and seat. This turned out to be true as his previous owner gave me his bitless bride and I have now had a new bitless bridle fitted for him. He is going to be amazing and has all the good parts of his Welsh D and Arab cross, but he needs a methodical approach.

Ten months on, he is making slow, steady progress and is growing hugely in confidence. Cheryl told me that Zing likes open spaces; this is true as he is still wary of going into a stable, preferring the open field. He clenches his jaw when he is worried – I see this often when he learns a new task, as he pulls his lower lip in. As he is sensitive across his nose, I am careful when asking him to turn left or right, not to pull on the reins but to guide with my legs. He is very attuned to my voice and dials into it. Zing looks flashy, and with good nutrition, teeth and back checked and a routine, he is certainly growing into himself. He feels well and truly settled in his own home – a lovely and happy horse.

I found both readings exceptionally intuitive. Cheryl has helped me to understand both horses' personalities and adapt my own behaviour to suit theirs. I loved hearing about their feelings; Zing telling me he would like to go cross-country some day and Dior saying that we get on well. The bond that has been built between us cannot be underestimated thanks to the insight I had through Cheryl.

I look forward to having a follow-up reading so that I can reaffirm how they feel and make sure I am doing the right thing for them.

Chumley, Santos and Matilda – Jenny Jones

I have three horses: Chumley, Santos and Matilda. Chumley is a nine-year-old, rescued, spotty Dartmoor hill pony, who's

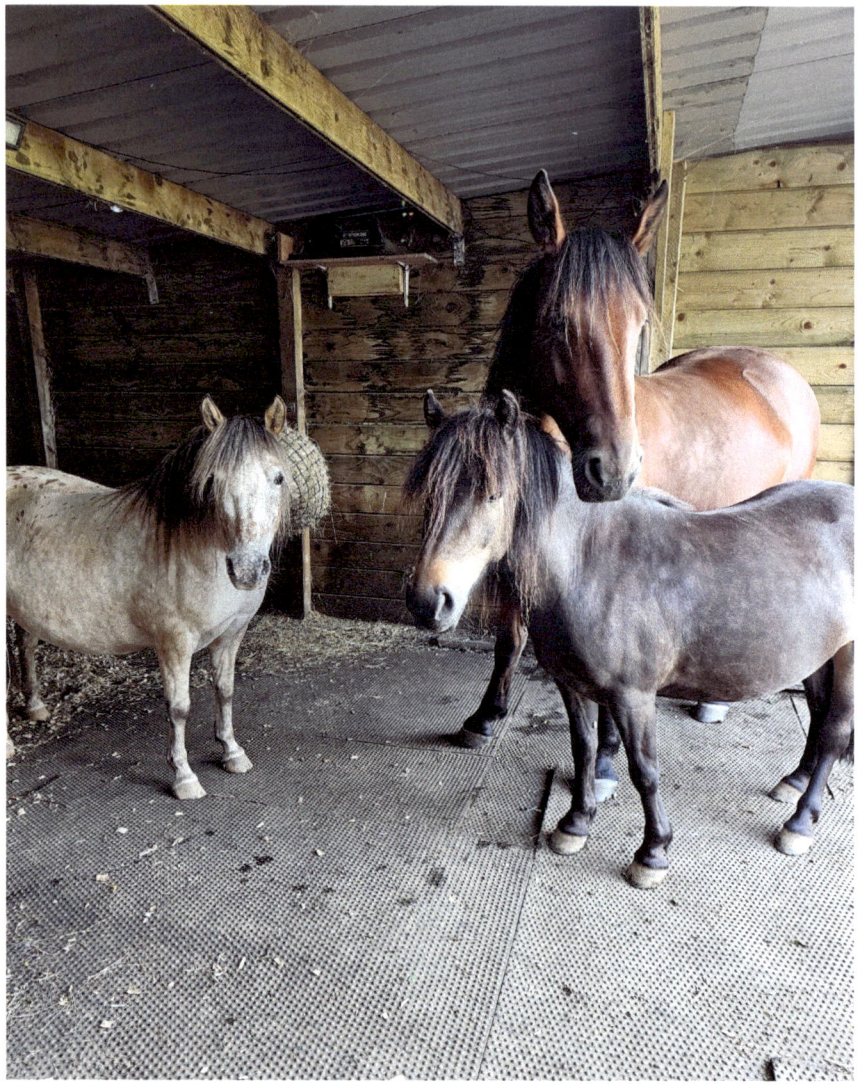

Chumley, Matilda and Santos. (Jenny Jones)

around 11.2hh; Santos is a three-year-old, another rescue, dark bay Dartmoor hill pony, who's approximately 11hh; Matilda is a two-year-old, bay Cluffolk (Mum is a Cleveland Bay, Dad is a Suffolk Punch), approximately 15.3hh.

There weren't any serious problems that I wanted help with, however, a lot of changes had happened over the last couple of years with the ponies – the loss of one, and two new additions for Chumley. I also knew Chumley was a troubled soul; my feeling was that she'd had quite a traumatic start to life, and she was hanging on to a lot of stress, so I wanted some guidance on how she wanted me to help her. I'd been doing what I felt was helping and had made progress, but there was clearly something else she needed.

Chumley had a poor start in life, and when she came to me, she was very aloof, and wasn't very interested in communicating with me. Her body felt very tense all the time, she hated being touched, and she had weight issues, with a thick cresty neck and fat pads in the usual places. She seemed unhappy, pulling faces, and not wanting to interact with others very much, which concerned me. I'd also been made aware of a fall she'd had in the field as a baby, with a suspected sacroiliac injury, which was never looked at or treated. This became very apparent to me when I did some exercise with her on the lunge to help with her weight loss, and after a few weeks, she became quite stiff behind. I've had her treated with my Zone Technique practitioner, who has helped her immensely.

I heard about Cheryl via social media, where people had put up posts asking for an animal communicator for their horse, and out of interest, I looked through the comments to see who was being recommended. From there, I came across Gemini Animal Communication, had a look at Cheryl's page and read her reviews. They certainly speak for themselves. I was drawn to her and felt that she was definitely the one who was going to help us.

My horses are my life, and I do absolutely everything I can to make sure they're kept to the very best of my care, knowledge, and experience and, most importantly, that they're happy and healthy. I'm always researching and studying, wanting to learn more all the time, so that I can do better. Their happiness is all I care about, and as much as I feel that my horses are happy, healthy and that I'm communicating with them and listening to them as far as possible, for me, to be able to speak with someone who could communicate with them on that higher level and get the feedback from them, fill in the gaps that I'm missing, so that I can be a better 'mum', was the thing I wanted to be able to do for my ponies. I wanted to give them a voice to let me know how I'm doing.

Cheryl and I had a consultation over the phone on 3 February 2023. I had a consultation with all three of them, as they're my herd, and I wanted to know what was happening between us, and also the relationship between them all. I just want to add here that I'd not mentioned a single thing about any of my horses to Cheryl, prior to this call.

The consultation started with her looking through all three eyes, saying their names accordingly. When she mentioned Matilda, I had a good laugh, as her words were, 'Matilda, ah Matilda, we'll come to her last, we need to have a few words with her!' And of course, she was absolutely spot-on! I'll come to her later.

We talked about Chumley first, as she was the one who I really feel needed the most help. She described Chumley with the most unbelievable accuracy. She said about Chumley having trust issues from long ago, and how it takes her such a long time to build trust in anyone. This, of course, is exactly what I'd been experiencing. She spoke about pain she was experiencing on her near-side, in front of the wither, across to the off-side shoulder and down into her pectoral muscle and scapula. She asked, 'Who's the big man with the beard?'

'That's my Zone Technique practitioner who's been treating her,' I replied.

Cheryl told me from Chum, 'I don't like him!'

It turns out that it wasn't anything personal – it's not that she didn't like him per se, she was very grateful for the good work he's done on her. What she didn't like about him was that he wasn't very friendly. Chum is very special and wants to be treated in a certain way. When he came to treat her, he went straight in and started with her, and she really didn't like it. She wants an introduction, the pleasantries, and to be asked if she's happy to be treated.

I asked if Chum had Equine Metabolic Syndrome (EMS) or Cushing's disease and she said no, which is great, as it confirmed what I felt. Cheryl said she could do with some liver and hindgut support; cow parsley was a good suggestion for this. Thankfully her chest and heart are both good and healthy. She also mentioned that her feet are a lot better now, too, which they are, they're looking great. She advised on getting some essential oils and offering them to her, to help with various things, which I have, and I do offer them to her randomly to see what she wants and needs, when she feels she needs it.

I got quite emotional when she said that Chum wants to be included more in everything, which was so lovely to hear. I've made a point of giving her kisses and cuddles, when she offers them to me of course! I've been working on her shoulder muscles and manipulating the trigger points in her pectoral muscles to help release her shoulder, which she really enjoys.

Overall, Chum has become relaxed, happier in herself, and interacts a lot more with me and the other two horses. I still don't force her to do anything, I always make a big fuss of her when I'm doing her feet, or if she's looking particularly happy I'll go and make a big fuss of her and let her know how much she's loved. She feels softer to touch and doesn't flinch when I touch her. She really has learnt to trust me now. Cheryl asked me if there was anything that I wanted to ask Chum.

I couldn't think of anything specifically, as I'd taken in so much information, so I asked her if there was anything Chum wanted to tell or ask me. Her reply brought tears to my eyes. She said, 'Chum wants you to know that your ability to listen is appreciated by them all, but mostly by her.'

It really melted my heart, knowing that she's recognised my effort in trying hard to listen to her, and meet her needs. She's such a beautiful soul and her issues are not her fault. It's just she's never had anyone take the time to listen to her.

Santos, dear little Santos. He's worth his weight in gold, was the first thing Cheryl said to me – and he is. I ended up looking for another companion for Chum, as I had very suddenly lost Vico, my Dutch warmblood. Although I had the foal in the pipeline, still in her mum's tummy, losing Vico was never in the plan. Matilda was born exactly one week before I lost him, so with six months before she was going to arrive, I wasn't prepared to leave Chum on her own for that time.

I found Santos at a lovely little rescue centre in Devon and chose him from around twenty-five others; I wish I could have taken them all! But I was thinking about a companion for Chumley, and who she would have chosen. Thankfully, I got it right.

When we brought him down to meet her, her little face lit up. She was absolutely delighted with him, and they were grooming each other within minutes. I cried with joy; I was so happy for her.

Santos's motto is 'Every day is the best day of my life.' And it truly is. He is just in love with life. Cheryl continued that he loves the sheep, he can't quite work out what they are, he knows they're not horses, but they fascinate him (I cross-graze my pet sheep with my horses, but Cheryl didn't know this). She then said, 'Who's the little person? He loves her.'

I laughed so hard! I have a lovely young girl who helps me muck out a few mornings a week, and she happens to be only 4ft 9in. When she's there, Santos just goes and stands with her while she's mucking out, hanging around and generally making a nuisance of himself. He loves everything about life, he's such a happy soul. Cheryl said he also adores my partner, who's not a horsey person, but he does enjoy a cuddle with Santos because he's calm and small.

Cheryl spoke quite clearly about Santos and the role he plays between Chum and Matilda. As two girls, they're bound to have their disagreements. Well, dear little Santos feels it's his job to keep the peace between them and he fulfils this role perfectly. When they're all feeding off one hay net, or they're all grazing together, nine times of out of ten, it'll be Chum, Santos, Matilda. He purposefully puts himself in the middle.

Santos will push his luck, because life is just a game for him. Cheryl said that he's forgotten all about his poor history and the start he had in life, he doesn't think about it any more. I didn't have any concerns with Santos, or his health particularly – all I wanted to know from him was that he was happy and healthy. Again, Cheryl asked me if I wanted to ask him anything, and I said the same as I did for Chum, 'What would he like to tell or ask me?'

She replied, 'Santos wants you to know that he feels his job is full-time and he doesn't need any distractions!' So, this is relating to being the peacemaker between the other two. He does this so well, and if things do get 'heated' in any way, he really does step in and diffuse the situation. He just wants peace and harmony in the camp. He lives every day like it's the best day of his life and wants the others to do the same.

Last, but by no means least, we came to Matilda. Quite honestly, I don't know where to start! To give a little background, Matilda was always very bold and confident from the moment she was born. She had pretty much weaned herself at four months and was wandering off doing her own thing all the time. I went to see her at two months and again at four months, and on both visits, I could clearly see how special she was.

Going back to Cheryl's words about her, she said she knows just how well she's bred and how special she is. She also knows how much I love her. Cheryl asked me what my plan was with her in her riding career, and I said that I was going to do a bit of everything and see what she enjoys the most.

'Jumping,' she replied. 'She wants to jump!' Of course, that's absolutely fine with me.

Cheryl went on to talk about Matilda and Chumley's relationship. Matilda respects Chum, she is aware of her ability to double-barrel out the back end and is very wary around her. She will always move out of Chum's way. Chum, to be fair, doesn't mince her words either, she makes herself very clear when she's not happy. Although Matilda knows damn well she's so much bigger than Chum, and that she could easily win the fight, she just allows Chum to have her place without any arguments. She wants peace and just lets it go.

Cheryl then mentioned that Matilda doesn't like being micromanaged. I know exactly what she means! In the first year, to start the correct education, I used a halter to teach her to stand politely to have her feet picked out, and anything else that I needed to do. Cheryl specifically mentioned that she said she didn't like it. With all three of them, I can do their feet, treat anything if needed, groom, worm, whatever it is, and I can do it all at liberty. As long as I show Matilda what I'm doing and explain it to her verbally, she will happily stand there and let me do it. If I don't show her that respect, she'll walk away. She's so funny. I started doing everything at liberty because to get the headcollar, put it on, lead them to a specific place etc., it all takes a lot more time. It's just so much easier to walk over to them and do it.

Cheryl advised me that she will push boundaries. No surprises there! She will try, however, I do kindly correct her if she oversteps the mark. She looks very sorry for herself when she knows she's done wrong. Despite her size, she is only two and still very much a baby, and she's not doing anything that any young horse wouldn't do. She's learning all the time and I'm learning with her, so we're learning together.

Cheryl gave me some very useful information to help when working with Matilda. She said to visualise what I want her to do (I'm still getting into the habit of using the visualisation technique). She has an exceptionally low boredom threshold, so all training has to be little and often. She learns so quickly, and if you just keep repeating the same thing, she'll just tell you she's had enough!

Cheryl also gave me some advice for when I do back her and start her riding career. It was back to micromanagement again. She said, whatever you do, don't override her. Don't force her, or try and control everything, let her do her job, as she'll know what she's doing. You know what? I can absolutely believe that, just by the way she is now. Cheryl said if anyone else rides her (highly unlikely!) and they start riding with their ego and trying to do fancy things with her, then it's time to make a cup of tea, pull up a chair and get your video rolling, because within five minutes of them riding her like this, she will tell them exactly what she thinks, and they will end up eating dirt. We had a good laugh about this; it was so amazing to chat with someone who knows exactly what she's like. The fact that Cheryl had never even met her is just truly remarkable.

To finish, as with the other two, she asked me if there was anything I wanted to ask Matilda. My reply was the same, what would she like me to know?

Cheryl told me 'Matilda feels she made her point and feels she has nothing further to add!'

My relationship with Chumley, Santos and Matilda, and the relationship between them, has got much more relaxed, with a deeper understanding of each other. Chumley's tightness and tension in her body has softened; she's still grumpy when she's in season, but I can understand that. She's so much happier in life, with me, the others, and our little herd set-up. There's still a way to go with her, and I'll keep working with her to really allow her to let go of all the previous stresses she's been hanging on to.

Santos will always be Santos, he'll never change. If he's quiet, I definitely know there's something not right! He's always happy, smiling (he loves smiling at everyone) and just goes with the flow, keeping the peace between the other two if needed, and as long as he's got them, and me, he doesn't care.

As Matilda is going to be my next riding horse, and I'm doing it all myself, I'm really focusing on our relationship; building trust and respect, which works both ways, and trying to get a really deep level of understanding of each other. These last few months, I've really noticed a difference in our connection, there are times where she does know what I would like her to do, and all I've done is to think about it. She's become so giving, tries her heart out to please, and will try and get away with naughty things occasionally! She's two years old, so what can you expect?

I keep my horses in the most natural environment I possibly can, they live out 24/7 on a track, with access to a huge shelter, ad lib hay, they can play, groom, and socialise whenever they want. I allow them to be horses and to express themselves.

I listen very intently to what they're telling me. I see them as my greatest teachers, after all, they're the experts at being horses and knowing what they need. My job is to watch, listen, and sit peacefully in those silent conversations we have between us, and never stop learning.

I feel so blessed to have found Cheryl, and so do my horses, I'm sure. To have someone who can communicate on that level with our animals, is possibly the greatest gift a true animal lover could wish for. I'm so grateful that I have this support and guidance whenever I need it, and with Matilda being such a strong character, I now know that everything is going to be just fine.

I'll be having regular sessions with Cheryl; I like to have two a year, to keep on top of things and make sure that I'm not missing anything. It's also really important for me that my horses have their voices heard and are able to get across what they want to say. This is their health and happiness, and as owners, it's our responsibility to make sure that we're providing what they need on an individual basis, and as a herd.

I love our consultations with Cheryl, they make me laugh, cry, and give me so much to think about, and also the reassurance that we're doing okay. In fact, not just okay, but really good! Thank you, Cheryl.

Jamal – Richard Kyle Hayes

I've worked with Cheryl on so many horses that it was hard to even remember which ones she has helped and how! I've gone with Jamal's story, because this amazing horse was my heart horse.

I saw a photo of him advertised and that was it, I knew I had to have him. I told my wife, who rolled her eyes; me wanting to buy horses I have instantly fallen in love with is a

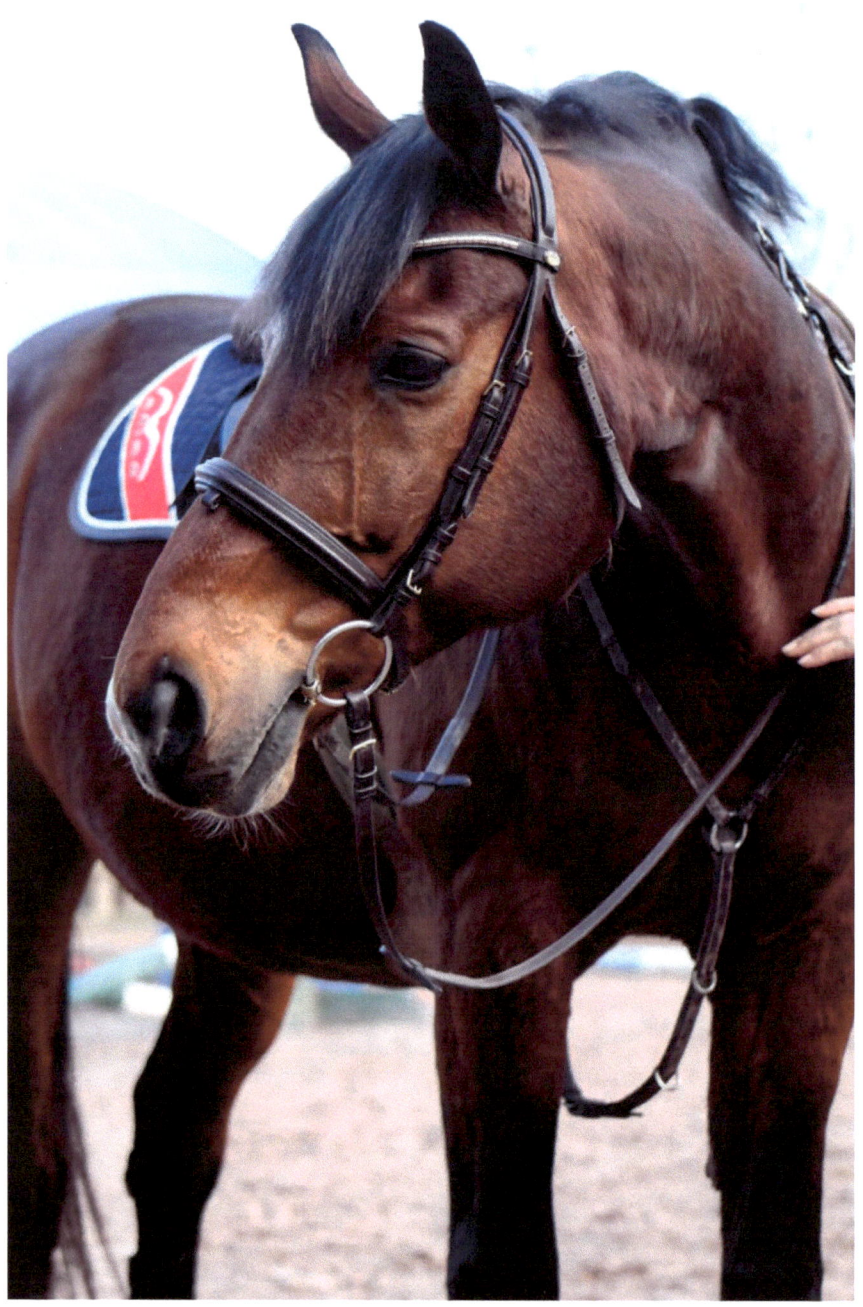

Jamal. (Richard Kyle Hayes)

regular occurrence! But this one was different. He was much older than those I usually went for, being nineteen when I bought him, but I was thinking he would be perfect for me to use as a coaching horse being that little bit older, and maybe steadier. He was utterly perfect.

Jamal was a complex horse, he was a Selle Français who had previously been an international top-level competition horse, and he certainly was a character. At a dressage competition we once attended, the judge was forced to say, 'We don't need the levade, thank you,' as Jamal sat himself down during the test!

He was very particular about his tack, and I had spent far more money than I should have, trying to find a saddle that was comfortable for him. I had heard about Cheryl and thought that I should give it a go, rather than spending any more money on tack that still didn't fit.

I was half-expecting a strange, witchy character with voodoo beads and bangles, so I was very surprised when Cheryl appeared to be absolutely normal! She talked me through everything about Jamal that she shouldn't have known – for example, I had recently bought a Stubben bridle, but had been too self-conscious to put Jamal in it because I was so sure he'd look like a character from *Star Trek*! No one knew I had bought that bridle, except Jamal, of course. Cheryl told me, 'That brown bridle you've got in the tack room, that's the one. It won't look *Star Trek*-y.'

She had never seen this bridle, I had not told her about it, but true to form this ended up being the one that worked best for Jamal.

Ever since then, I have worked with Cheryl on many horses, and I've been amazed every single time. Talking to Cheryl is like getting a warm hug, and to hear, through her, all the things that you can't hear your horses saying, is amazing.

And, just in case you were doubting this woman's abilities, let me tell you about when Jamal died. I had been coming back from an equine fair in Ireland, and as I came closer to home, I had a sick feeling in my stomach, and I knew there was something wrong with Jamal. I even called my wife to meet me at the field to check on him. When we got there, he had suffered some sort of catastrophic accident and his leg was completely shattered. I had to call the vet and have Jamal put down within twenty minutes of being home.

I was utterly devastated, but I never told Cheryl. We were booked in for another consultation for a different horse, and I still hadn't told her. I still found it painful to talk about, but I think a small part of me wanted to test her. Anyway, the time came; she phoned and we exchanged pleasantries. Then she suddenly stopped mid-sentence, and said, 'Oh Kyle, why didn't you tell me?' She knew. The connection this woman has to horses is something truly special and I am so grateful to her for helping my horses.

Clooney – Claudia Faraday

I bought Clooney being fully aware of his medical history and knowing that he had had kissing spines. I knew what I was getting myself into. I am an equine physiotherapist, so I do have a lot of experience with treating horses, and I knew that this horse would be a challenge. I hoped that my experience as a physio would help with Clooney's issues. I brought him home when he was rising six, he is now seven and still going strong, but we've been through a lot in the meantime.

Despite spending thousands with the vet, and my own physio experience, I couldn't find where Clooney's pain was and neither could the vet. All our efforts appeared to be in

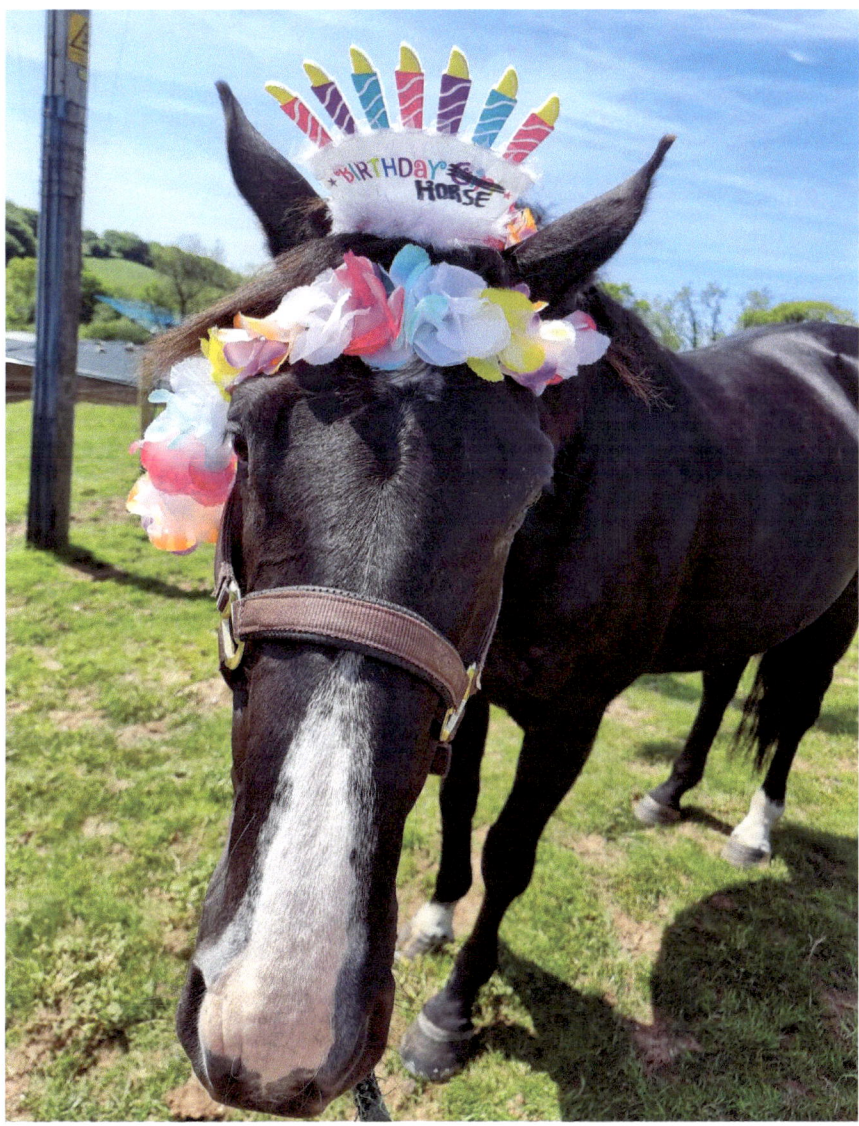

Clooney. (Claudia Faraday)

vain, and in desperation and heartbreak, it was arranged to have Clooney put to sleep in February 2022. Enter Cheryl.

She told me that Clooney had kidney strain and nerve pain in his face – this correlated to my experiences tacking him up – and she advised a selection of natural remedies and oils to treat his problems. Clooney is now doing extremely well, riding out and happy, and about as far from being put down as he could possibly be.

Interestingly, Cheryl appears to be able to 'read' people as well. She came to see another mare of mine one day and described her personality to a tee – she was angry, grumpy and feeling frustrated because she wanted to do more, and I wasn't giving her enough. Then Cheryl started to say that the mare was suffering sacroiliac pain and for the first time I thought 'She's wrong.' I pushed myself away from the door that I had been leaning on – resting myself because of my sacroiliac pain – and asked if she was sure. Cheryl put her hand on my arm then laughed and threw me out of the stable – she'd been accidentally 'reading' me!

When I was losing my way, Cheryl helped me by opening other doors for me to look through, the type that neither the vet nor I even knew existed. She's been my cheerleader (though I call her a witch to her face!) and has helped me and my horses tremendously. My job is intensely scientific; you have to know which part of the anatomy you are dealing with, it's all written down and proven and easy to make sense of – but you have to remain open-minded with everything in this world, and especially with horses.

I started looking for other horses when it seemed unlikely that Clooney would ever be ridden again. I found one I liked the look of, found out everything about him – including his health issues – and then sent a picture of his eye to Cheryl. There would be no way she could have found out about the diagnosis of this horse, but she knew anyway – from looking at a picture of an eye. You can't really make this stuff up, can you?

Hertog – Marika Mays

My own horse that Cheryl saw was the stunning Hertog, a 17hh chestnut Gelderlander and an enormous character. I owned him for four years, from getting him started at the age of four, until a horrific and rapid colic took him from me at just eight.

About two years into owning him I had Cheryl out, as he was a wonderful albeit cheeky playful boy, but he just would not go forward under saddle. He loved to go out hacking (not wanting to go home after) and to go in the school, but he refused to work enough to ever get sweaty. I worked through all I knew as a therapist and couldn't find a physical cause or any hint of lameness – he was just sore because of walking on stony ground (he was barefoot).

Before contacting the vet with no information to guide their investigations, it was time to get Cheryl in. We had a wonderful hour with her chatting about his health, life and humorous stories. I discovered that he was much happier with saddle and bridle changes and had nothing to complain about there.

He loves to play in the school but has no desire to work. Cheryl described him aptly as a 'Kevin the Teenager'. If there was no fun, there was no point! I asked about when I got very insistent on pushing him forward and did that worry or scare him? He was apparently laughing, saying that I 'hit like a fly' and that I felt guilty after he got his way more. That was a real eye-opener, as I had only owned horses before who had experienced some prior abuse and were highly sensitive mares – he was by contrast a bit of a thug and enjoyed a bit of physicality.

Cheryl's advice was to be very black and white with him moving forward, and to keep things as fun as possible. It was lovely to hear he was devoted to me from the moment we met and I felt very lucky.

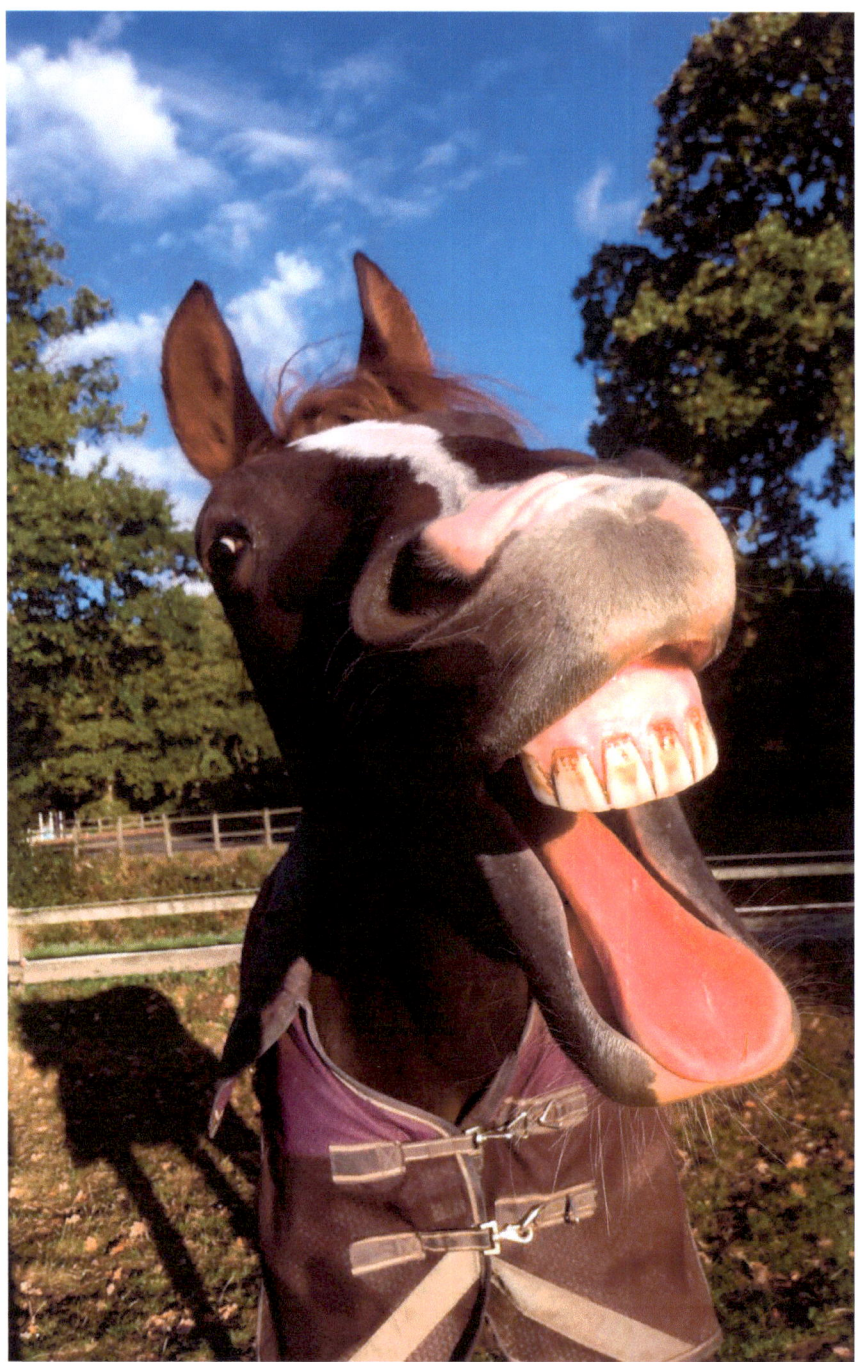

Hertog. (Marika Mays)

I felt guilty when Hertog explained his distress after our first meeting, when I didn't take him straight home or tell him mind-to-mind what I would do. He told his horse buddies that he'd found his owner and was going off, but nothing happened for a week, and he became very sad. I now make more effort with horses to keep them in the loop, even if it's over the brainwaves when I can't be there in person with them.

Hertog talked about what therapies and techniques he loved from me, and which ones he thought were ineffective. He also gossiped about other horses on the yard and his jealousy over who was in which field. At this point his language was fitting for a Kevin the Teenager, i.e. lots of colourful swearing! When asked about where he picked up the swearing, he had this beyond excited, gossipy look on his face as he reported on another livery owner – who was, funnily enough, on their last warning for swearing in the yard!

I loved the validation Cheryl gave of his personality, which she nailed. He had some very odd behaviours that I made no mention of to her myself. This included how much he loved to stand on things, throw objects at people for a laugh, hold water in his mouth to drop down my wellies or my trousers if I bent over, and just playing with water generally. He also told her how much he detested water on his back; he would throw himself against the stable walls violently if he'd got a wet back when riding, caught a shower in the field without a rug on, or had a rare bath. You can see what a character he was.

After Cheryl's advice I did change my approach to riding, and became more determined, and I suppose dominant, but I tried to keep things fun. He did improve in the school but only moderately. Getting sweaty and working hard just wasn't for him, but at least I wasn't worried that I was missing some underlying pain and being cruel by asking him to work.

It gave me peace of mind and it was nice to confirm that his idea of rough play with me was because he was having fun with a buddy, and not from anger, so I just channelled that energy into fun tasks and more human-friendly forms of play.

So how did I know about Cheryl? Well, this was through my training in JENT (Jenkins Equine Neurophysiologic Therapy) with Dianne Jenkins. Stories of this amazing communicator and some of the information gleaned from her on certain horses arose many times during my training. It wasn't until I needed help with Hertog that I first thought to try Cheryl out myself and despite working with energy in some weird and wonderful ways, I still had some reservations on how much I could get from it.

Within five minutes of us meeting her I had no reservations any longer. The chat from Hertog was detailed, spot-on and could never have been known from any inauthentic means or 'good guesswork' like some critics suggest. Cheryl has a wonderful gift.

She worked on other horses on the yard who I was treating and who had very different personalities and physical problems, and I was so impressed with her accuracy and insight with them, too.

As a therapist I have had some rare but delightful sessions where she is simultaneously working on the same group of horses. I wish this was possible regularly, especially with atypical cases or horses showing signs of emotional trauma.

On one occasion I had done several sessions on a warmblood who pulled angry faces when I was approaching certain techniques on his hind end, so I would defer those for when he showed he was ready (self-preservation, and because I like to feel the horse has autonomy in their treatment). When Cheryl was treating the adjoining horse, she relayed to me that the horse I was working on was worried but wanted me to do it anyway and would keep me safe. The technique was done without issue and the horse said it was much improved after. Without Cheryl there, how long would it have been before I had got that done?

In another instance working on a warmblood, Cheryl was able to confirm my instincts with some hidden pain locations that didn't fit exactly with expectations. One of these was his headaches. I was able to play with some different techniques for loosening muscles around the head with live feedback from Cheryl on what he felt with each one and the moment the tension causing the headache released. What a privilege! I also work on people and it's great to have that live feedback for when you locate the relevant trigger point in a muscle that is causing that specific headache – it's a very particular feeling. When working with horses, it is wonderful to have someone there who can tell me, through them, when I've got it right.

I have many clients who use Cheryl, but most of them can't or don't tie us in together. While together is ideal, that doesn't diminish how beneficial it is to hear Cheryl's conversations with my horsey clients on what techniques they like most, that they perhaps asked for me to come again, where they say they feel pain, etc.

I always worry that my horses will complain about me or tell Cheryl the stupid stuff I do. Will they laugh about when I fell over in the school during lungeing? Do they think I'm being grumpy as I'm perimenopausal? But so far so good and if they say anything tactless, Cheryl keeps it to herself.

Sadly, I lost Hertog to a sudden, unexpected colic a week before Cheryl's second visit. Cheryl came out anyway and we were able to chat to him 'beyond the veil', using a photo of his face to help her connect. This session was hugely beneficial for me, as I was still in shock and deeply grieving this enormous, loving personality who brought me joy every day. There is always a measure of guilt and failure when you lose a horse traumatically. Did I do something to cause it? Did I miss some signs I should have understood?

Cheryl was able to reassure me that it was just one of those things. He hadn't felt any warning signs and it was just bad luck. Hertog hadn't wanted to leave me and I had felt his energy around me for many days, unlike previous horses who I felt moved on within minutes. Apparently an extremely old horse kept coming to guide him over the veil and got insistent. This would have been my first horse who I lost to old age at thirty-two and she really looked ancient by then. It was great to know she had come back to guide Hertog and would keep tabs on me, too, occasionally.

Hertog had some strong views on what he wanted me to do with the hair I kept from his tail. He said, 'None of that awful jewellery, please!' I was allowed to use some with a blue calcite crystal, which he wanted me to then use to develop my own communication skills in the future. Hertog also said it was great that he now wasn't held in by field boundaries, and he could go and complain to the horses in the field he preferred. He was a very dominant horse with a strong sense of his own worth.

There was no reduction in his personality beyond the veil. He had a lot to say about some of the horses I had been looking at to buy – how they were too small; how his tack and rugs wouldn't fit them. I didn't want to replace this shining star, but because once you have a horse-shaped hole, there's nothing else that can fill the void they leave.

Cheryl and I looked at pictures of one big Irish youngster who had caught my eye. Hertog didn't complain about him or say much at all, but Cheryl connected with Seamus and asked him how he felt about my plans, his health, and checked out his basic personality for me. He had lots of head pain he wanted help with and he was curious to try things with me, but she said he was stubborn and not used to following the guidance of humans; he very much thought for himself. I should have been warned! I met him a couple of days later and I love a challenge, so I got him. Cheryl is booked to come and meet him, as it has been a very difficult journey and, boy, does he have strong views!

I asked the universe to help me find a personality as big as my beloved Hertog's and someone who needed me. I should have been more precise with my request and specified someone calm who enjoyed looking after me and working hard in the school. Maybe in a couple of decades, after my time with Seamus.

I'm very lucky that Hertog still pops by on occasions to check in on me, and that my new boy has an equally large personality. I get a lot of love from my horses, which is lucky as I also get quite a number of demands and danger.

Hertog would love to be immortalised in print. He would find it very fitting as he is a very important soul, so I like to think he would approve of this.

Janni – Jude Smith

The first horse I had Cheryl out to read was my Friesian mare, Janni (you may know her as the 'Batman horse' from the image that went viral a few years ago). I bought her, having fallen in love with her and her beautiful Baroque style. She would be perfect for the dressage I loved. Well, I brought her home and I can only describe her as a complete psycho! I was unable to catch or tack her up for months at a time, and she really did not seem happy.

We eventually got past this and started working together under saddle; she was everything I could have wished for. She then

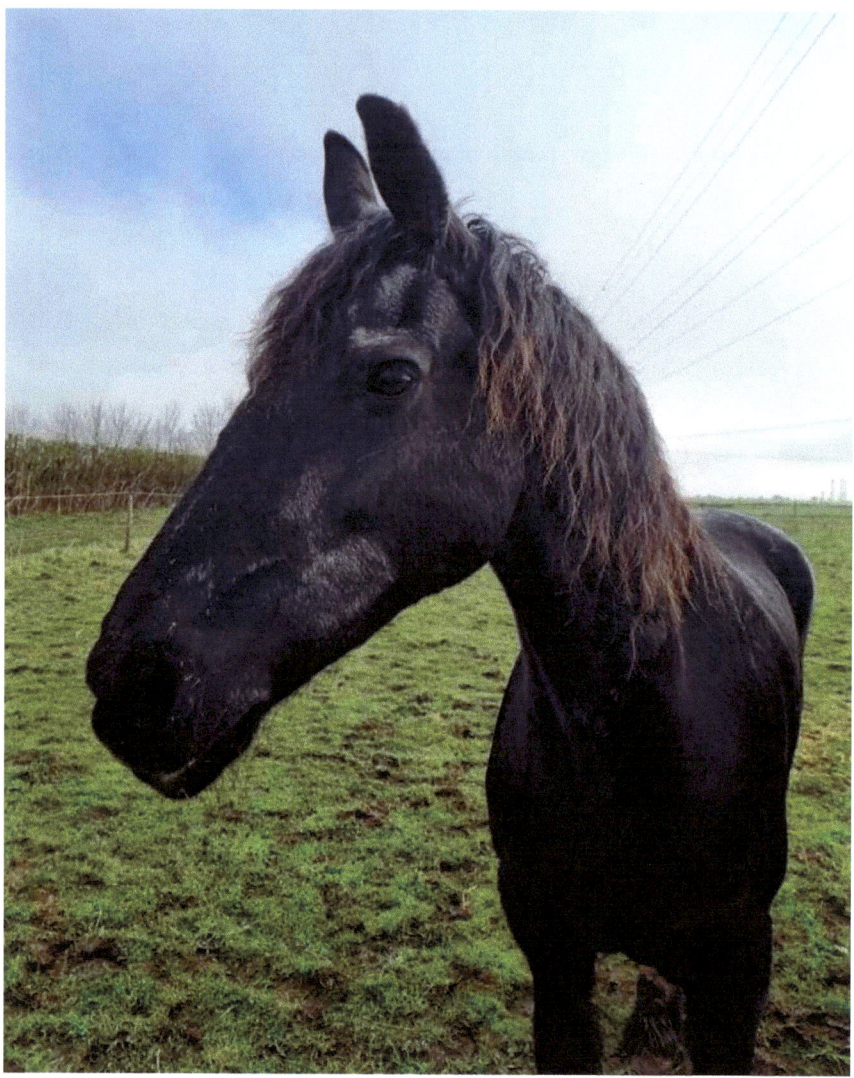

Janni. (Jude Smith)

suffered an injury in the field and obviously I called the vet out. She was diagnosed with a split in the meniscus of her stifle and the vet advised me that she would never be sound, never be pain free, and that the kindest thing I could do was to put her out of her misery. Well, we all trust our vets, don't we? But I couldn't bring myself to put an end to this beautiful horse's life.

With no other leads to follow, I was pretty desperate. I had seen some reviews for Cheryl's work and decided that I had nothing to lose, so I called her out to see Janni. She described things she should never have known about, like her temperament and personality; the fact that she'd had a foal removed from her the day before I first saw her, this explained the psychotic behaviour; and even a perfect physical description of her seller – whom Cheryl had never seen or heard of.

I was advised to put Janni on a turmeric supplement, and Cheryl told me, 'You will be cantering when the sun is high in the sky.'

So, Janni duly got her turmeric, and she stayed with me for another eight years. I never asked her to work for me in dressage again, but we happily hacked out regularly, and one day when she was feeling particularly relaxed and comfortable I gave her the reins and we had a glorious, exhilarating canter. It was only later that I remembered Cheryl's words about cantering when the sun was high in the sky – it was a hot, sunny July day.

I am so blown away by the fact that I could have blindly followed the vet's advice, and had my beautiful mare put down and missed out on almost a decade that we had left to spend together. Instead, I followed Cheryl's advice and I could not have been happier.

When it finally came time to say goodbye to Janni, she went very fast. I had bought another Friesian, Dex, to continue my dressage and showing career, and he proved to be a big personality. Cheryl has also helped immensely with him and it took a while before he was ready. I fully believe Janni waited for this, because within a couple of weeks of Dex arriving, Janni went right downhill. I started giving her bute, which she refused to eat, and she would stand at the top of the field, just staring into nothingness.

I wanted Cheryl's opinion that it was time to let her go, because there's nothing worse than doing the deed too early – as I had already learned from my earlier experiences with Janni. Cheryl never told me in words of one syllable to put Janni down, but she told me I was doing the right thing, which made it easier to let go.

Cheryl, despite my initial scepticism, has proved to be the most wonderful advocate for my horses – and I'm sure, countless other people's, too. She gives our horses a voice, and I feel it shows us owners a whole new dimension to our horses. They have a personality; they have feelings; they have words – being able to hear those words is such a special gift. I now recommend Cheryl to everyone I meet – provided they are open-minded enough!

Splash – Elizabeth Irwin

I found Cheryl through a friend who had reached out to her asking for help with her cats; this was the first time I had heard about someone who could 'speak' to horses. I had recently purchased a horse for my eleven-year-old son as a step up from his loan pony to his own horse. I live in Australia, had searched for the best part of a year and had travelled thousands of kilometres looking for the perfect one.

Splash, the one who I believed ticked all the right boxes, was vetted and risk assessed and found to be perfect, so I arranged to have him transported to us from Queensland. It was an eighteen-hour journey, which was planned over two days with regular stops for welfare. I'll come back to the journey later.

Within six weeks of owning Splash, we discovered that he was completely unrideable; even handling him required me to wear full safety gear – hat, body protector, the lot. Splash would panic, rear and lash out with his front feet – all in all,

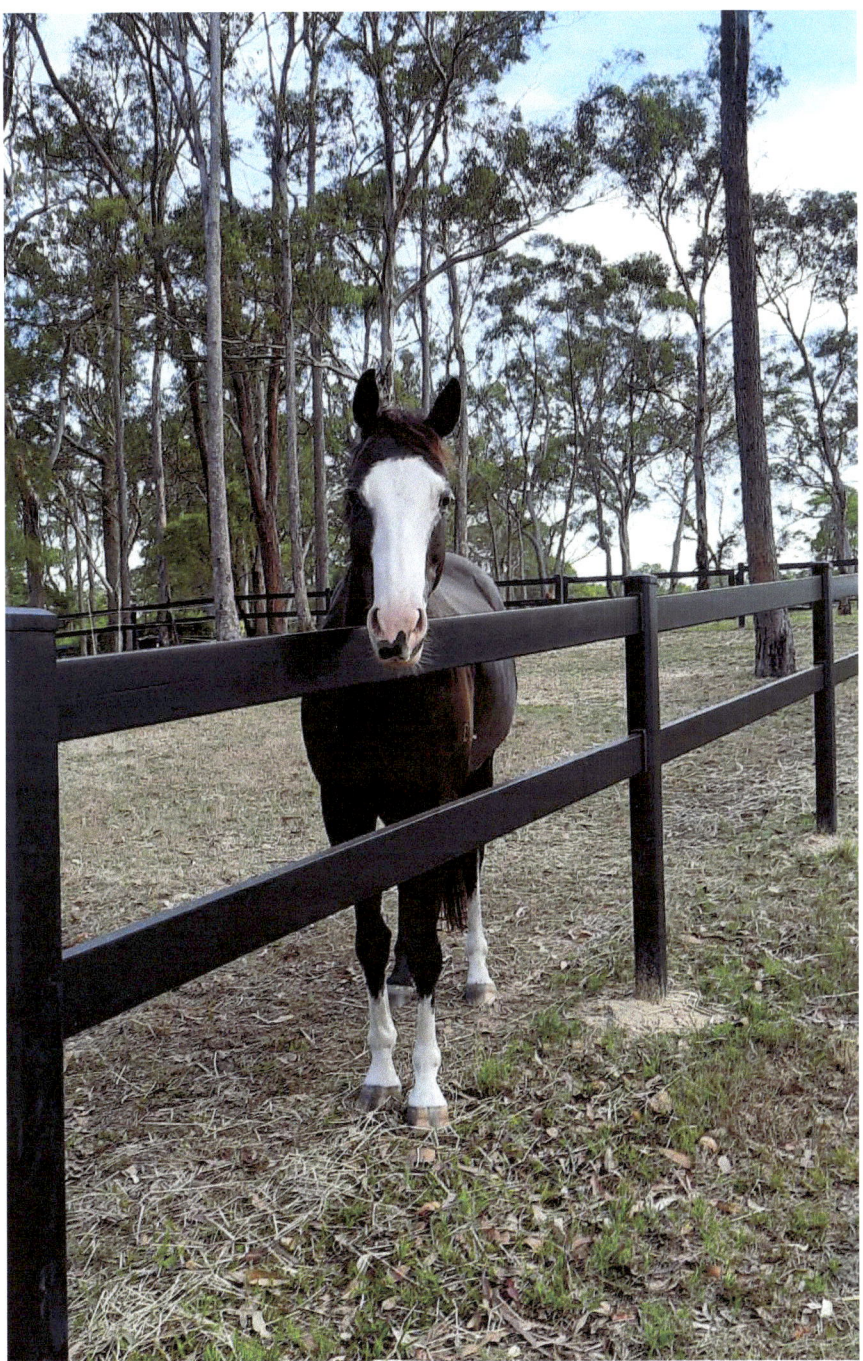

Splash. (Elizabeth Irwin)

he seemed like a dangerous horse and I was at a loss to know what to do. It took three months for my appointment with Cheryl to roll around and I was completely stuck.

When Cheryl tried to connect with Splash, she initially struggled because he was in so much pain. Because of our geographical differences it took us a while to find the right bodyworker to help Splash; we eventually settled on an Emmett therapy practitioner. Cheryl and Grantley worked together, and to this day it gives me chills to remember Cheryl being at home in the UK, on the phone to me and a bodyworker just outside Sydney, and Cheryl was able to describe exactly what was going on with Splash and what the bodyworker was doing.

Splash is still very much a work in progress; we are taking it very slowly and taking into account what Splash can handle, so it is small steps at a time. Splash is still not safe to ride, but he is working under saddle and getting stronger and more confident every day. Cheryl rightly suspected that Splash's issues were both physical and emotional, so we take care not to push it too hard.

My theory (although I am unable to prove this) is that Splash damaged himself during transit, which ended up not being the door-to-door service that I had asked for. Splash was dumped at a local transport depot with fifteen minutes' notice, and I had to travel to pick him up. This poor horse was frightened and confused, and his ears were not set straight on his head as they were before. I believe that he must have reared and smashed his head inside the original transport, which has led to nerve damage and explains the intense pain he was feeling.

We continue to work with Cheryl quarterly on improving life for Splash, and I strongly believe that with this amazing lady's help he will end up being happy, well-adjusted and a perfect pony. He certainly is much happier now that he knows this is his forever home, and we can take him out and about with us – without the need for every piece of protective gear under the sun!

Astro – Holly Wateridge

My horse, Astro, is a New Forest pony standing at 14.2hh. I'd had him for seven years when I called Cheryl in. Astro has a bone spavin in one hind leg and shivers in the other, and I wanted Cheryl to come out and see if he was comfortable with ridden work and if he felt happy with how we were managing his pain treatment. I am Astro's second owner and we went through hell and back in the first two years of having him, due to his old owner overworking him (which is what we thought had happened), but I also just wanted to find out more about his past.

Astro described himself as a 'pity purchase' for us, as his past wasn't that great, and for him to say he was happy with his life now and couldn't thank my family enough for taking him on was a delight to hear.

I heard amazing feedback about Cheryl from a yard friend as she'd called her out and, despite being sceptical about it, I went ahead and booked Cheryl to see Astro. Honestly, I've never looked back from having her out – to the point I had her come back when I moved yards so she could see if he was happy with the move. Apparently, Astro said it was, 'About time!'

Cheryl let me know all about his past – from what he could tell her anyway, as he said he has a memory like a fish. When she went through top to tail, he asked for his saddle to be checked, so I called out a new saddler and it turns out I had completely the wrong saddle on him. A new saddle was purchased and to say I have a different horse would be an understatement. He said he didn't like work on Cheryl's first

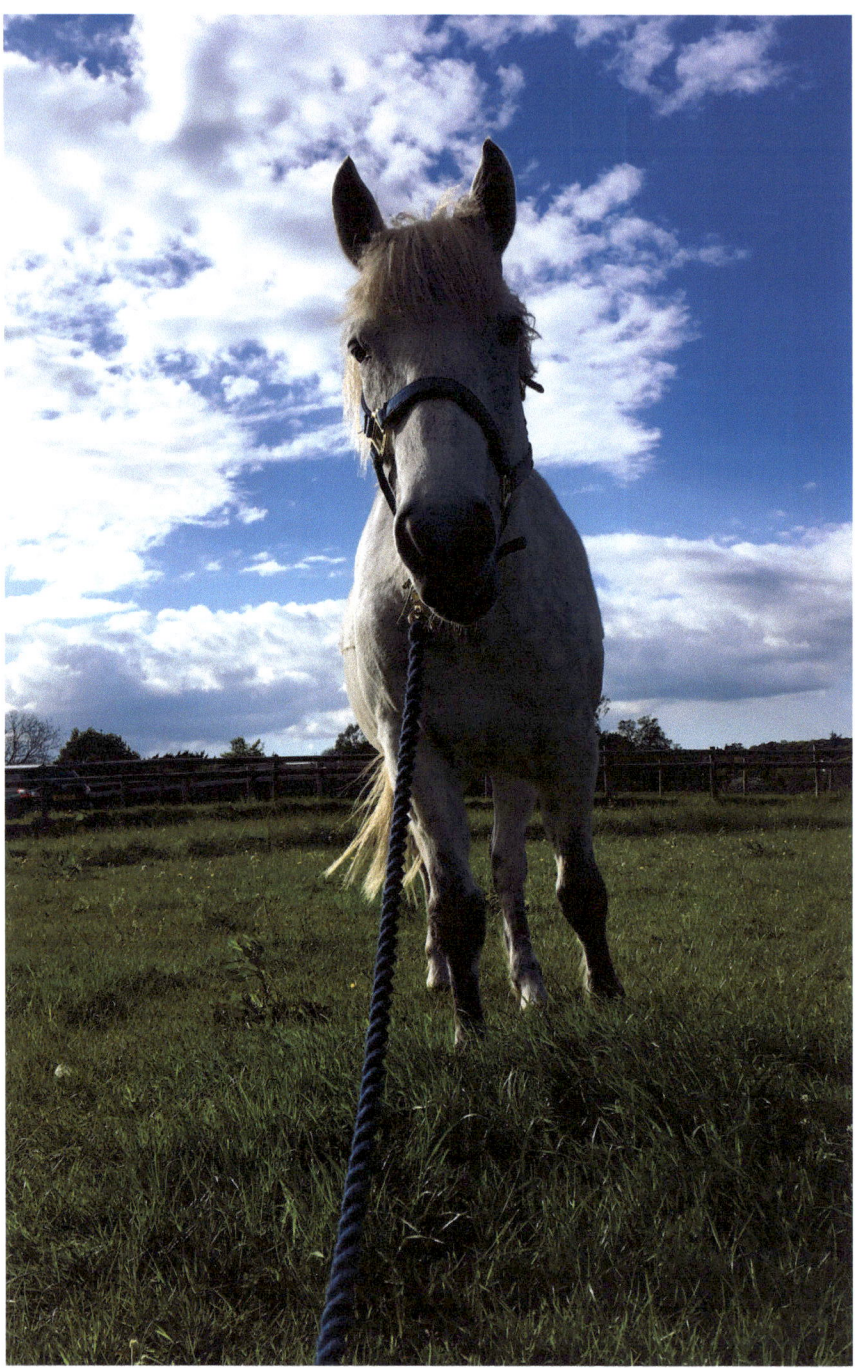

Astro. (Holly Wateridge)

visit, and on the second, after the new saddle, he said he now has joy to life. If you had told me seven years ago that Astro and I would be cantering and galloping through the woods, I would have told you 'No way!'

Astro and I now have such a happy relationship where he's happy to go out, happy with life and very comfortable in himself. He actually drags me out of the field, whereas before I felt like I was having to drag him. He also whinnies every time I go up to the field to see him, which is the loveliest thing, I now feel like he's pleased to see me.

Now I can ride Astro knowing he's not in pain and that he enjoys what he does and is able to go more than two paces. By the end of this year, we are hoping to go out in the trailer to some lessons, which I never thought I could do.

Not only has this helped Astro but it's given me such a confidence boost in my riding as I'm no longer scared of feeling that I'm hurting him.

Bee – Nicki Chenery

I bought Bee, now a 15.3hh four-year-old Hanoverian mare, unhandled and unbacked from a stud in West Sussex. I love dressage and I chose her because I wanted her to be my forever dressage horse.

As I started doing groundwork with her, it was apparent there were some things she was not happy with, especially when long-reining and anything touching her hind legs. I sent her to be backed at Connie Colfox's yard, and Connie worked a lot with her but always said there was an underlying issue that she couldn't put her finger on. I told Connie that I hoped she didn't think I was mad, but that I had heard of this lady who could probably help in a way that neither of us could, and when I said Cheryl's name she jumped at the chance. Connie

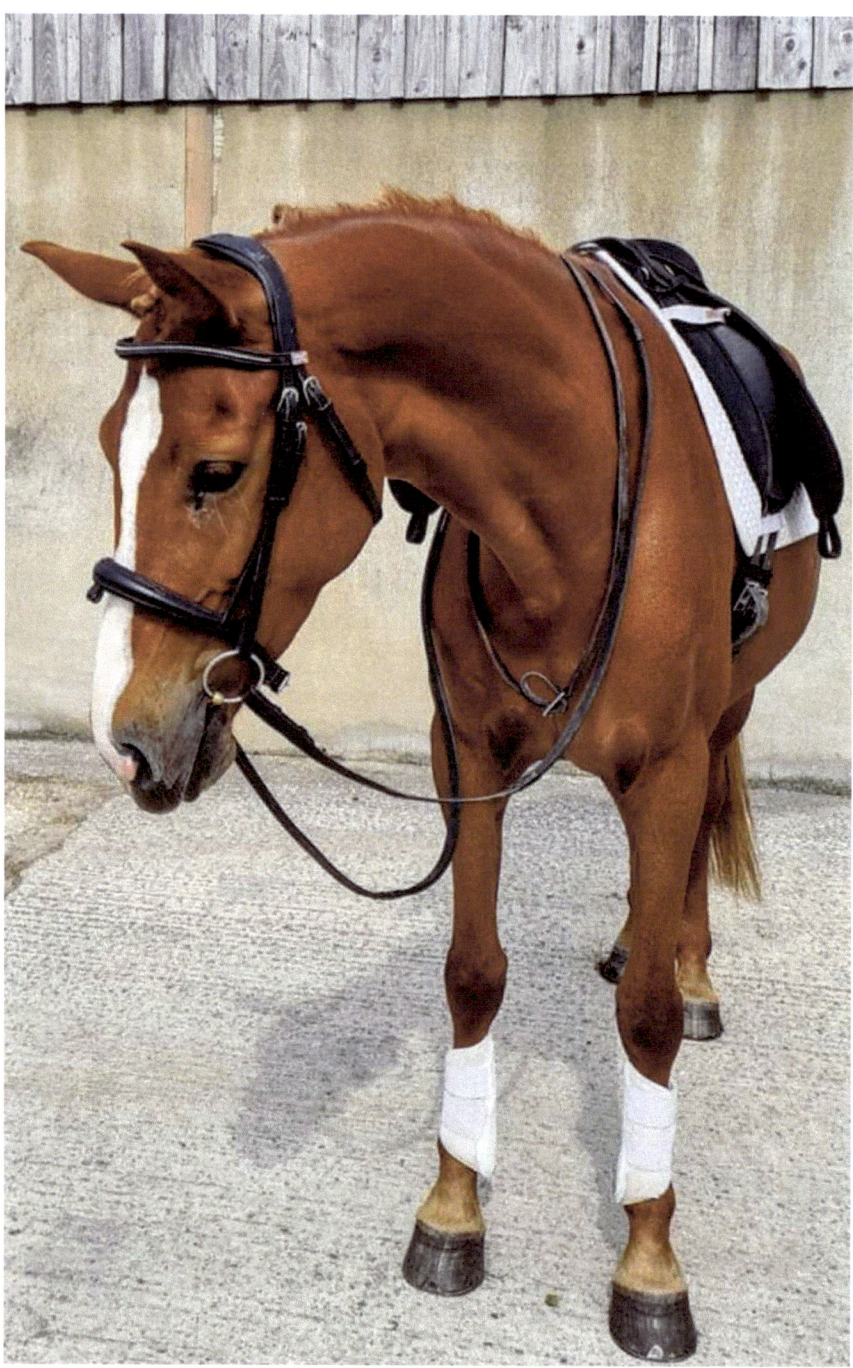

Bee. (Nicky Chenery)

had worked with Cheryl previously, so I knew if anyone would be able to help Bee it would be the two of them together.

Cheryl went to see Bee when she was at Connie's yard and Connie videoed it for me while Cheryl was on the phone to me. I could see how Bee was reacting to Cheryl, who mentioned some deep issues that would cause Bee to behave in the way she did, primarily Bee being in the same stable when her mum passed away. She said this had caused long-standing issues that we needed to work on with Bee.

Bee spent a few more weeks with Connie, and when I went and rode her there, I felt like we had turned a corner. I brought Bee back home and continued to work her in the same way and she seemed to be able to cope for a couple of weeks, but then something changed in her behaviour. I liaised with Cheryl a lot during this time – poor Cheryl must have been fed up with me, but she was the only one I could trust. It was decided that I should give Bee a couple of weeks off and then start again, it was a change of season and this affected her a lot, too.

When I started up groundwork again, I decided to long-rein her like Connie had and off we went. Something changed in Bee's brain and she decided to bolt off; unable to hold on to her I had to let her go. Once I finally caught her, she was in a terrible way. The emergency vets came, and she was around eight-tenths lame on her off-fore. They X-rayed and ultrasounded her, and all looked clear. Fast-forward two weeks and she was still as lame but after a bone scan of leg and shoulder, still no diagnosis was made.

I was trusting the science when I knew the only person that could help me, again, was Cheryl. I called her and said Bee had had an accident and she pinpointed each laceration, graze, bump, bruise that Bee had on each of her legs (it was a bad accident). I was shocked that she could tell me exactly where

Bee was hurting, especially since she had not witnessed the accident, or seen Bee since. She could not have known about the injuries and I was amazed. I knew that Cheryl could tell me what was wrong with that off-foreleg and when I asked her specifically about that leg, she said that Bee's foot was sore, there was a pulling somewhere. Cheryl said it was in the foot.

The following day I called the vet and asked what appeared on the bone scan of the foot? It turned out that they hadn't scanned the foot, so I asked them to come and do so. The vet asked me why the foot specifically, so I explained about Cheryl and told him that she had identified it while communicating with Bee to find out where she was hurting. The vet, of course, pooh-poohed this and said that nothing would be found.

Bee had that foot X-rayed and she had, in fact, fractured the wing of her pedal bone, exactly where Cheryl had said. Unfortunately, the prognosis was not good, and it was decided that Bee should be put to sleep, as it wasn't fair on her and her temperament, so the sad decision was made, but at least I could comfort myself with the fact that Bee was no longer in pain.

Hand on heart, my whole time with Bee would have been a lot different if I didn't have the expertise and help of Cheryl; there are no words to describe how special this lady is in so many ways. She continues to be my first port of call, in situations and has continued to help with my new horse in very different ways, too. People think I'm crazy sometimes, but the proof is in the results that Cheryl gets. I'm honestly not sure if I would be the horsewoman I am today if I had never met this wonderful lady.

Chilli – Krysta Moore

Chilli is a thoroughbred gelding who is ten years old. I've had him since he was four and he is a big boy at 16.1hh. Chilli and

Case Studies

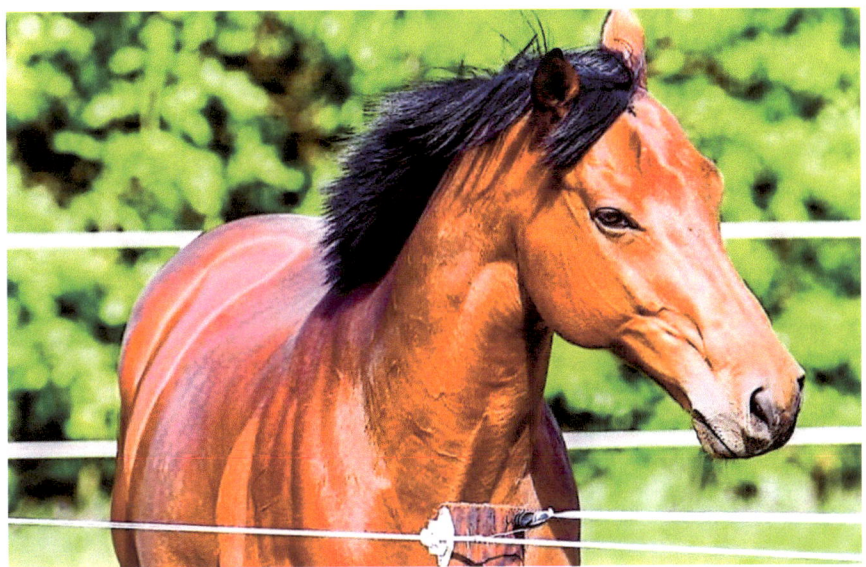

Chilli. (Krysta Moore)

I have been through a lot together and I've been very happy with him, however, we were having some issues with cross-country. He would be very unsure of himself and of me, and would go numb and unresponsive, which didn't do our performance any good. He just wasn't taking any guidance from me, and we were not progressing well and both becoming frustrated.

During our efforts at showjumping, I always felt that I was holding him back from his true potential, and I really wanted someone to help me out – however, it definitely wasn't a physical issue. I heard about Cheryl through a Facebook suggestion, and after reading a few of her reviews, I was pretty well-convinced. Needless to say, I organised a slot with Cheryl just as soon as I could.

Cheryl said that Chilli is so glad that I ride him, and that if it was anyone else that was trying to teach him a lesson he would, 'Dig my heels in and teach *them* a lesson.'

She said he may have some issues with his hocks, which was 100 per cent accurate, although I wasn't aware of this until Cheryl told me. I was never treating any specific area for him, but when he starting backing out of the trailer upon loading, and because Cheryl had drawn attention to his hocks, I brought him for a soundness assessment. Surprise, surprise, there was a problem and he has been medicated in that area ever since.

Meeting Cheryl has changed my relationship with Chilli; I know he is happy with me, and I understand him a lot more now. Our relationship, both our working one and general personal connection has changed positively, and I am so happy I came across Cheryl for her guidance. Chilli and I have gained trust in each other across the undulating ground of cross-country. It never occurred to me that he has an issue with not knowing what's on the other side of a jump or a mound or a hill, but we've worked on that and he's much better, and now listens to me and I guide him.

My experience with Cheryl was very positive, and I was very grateful to her for helping me to understand my horse better, and for allowing him his voice to express what was actually going on in his head.

Jive – Lou Loxton

Jive is a beautiful, sassy, Cremello, fourteen-year-old Welsh Section A, who I bought in 2023 as a pony for my little girl. She's still very young, so a lead rein/first pony is what I was looking for. Jive came from a loving family, but she had been pretty much left to her own devices as part of a herd, and I wanted to find out a little more about her past and her character.

I found Cheryl through Facebook and because of word of mouth – friends had used her in the past and had sung her praises. Jive was also a companion for my horse Mickey and I had also used Cheryl to 'check in' with Mickey, just to make

Case Studies

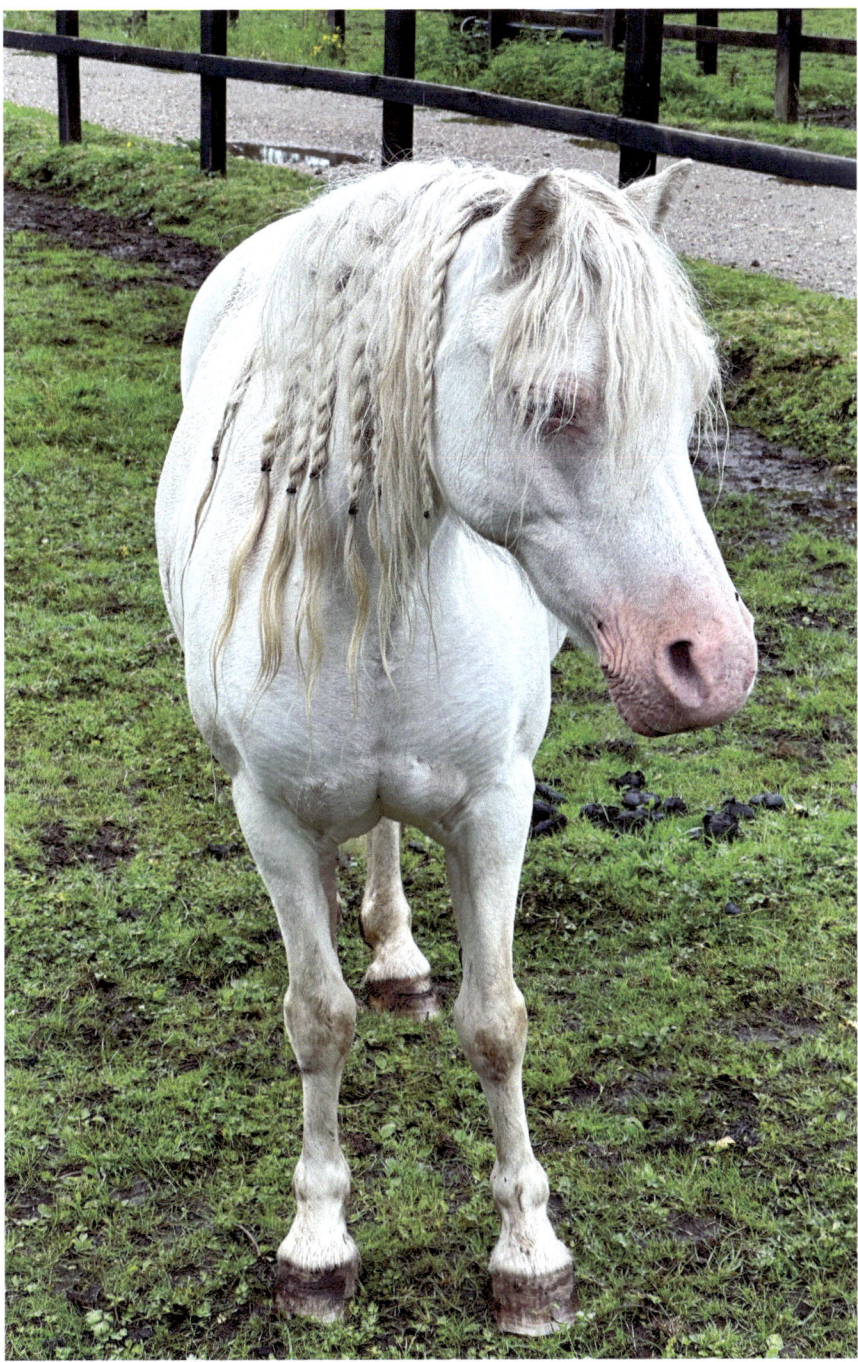

Jive. (Lou Loxton)

sure that he was happy, and I had been very impressed with her reading of him.

Jive was always meant to be a first-ridden pony for my little girl, but we have not done much with her, due to having to move yards and general life circumstances. Cheryl laughed when she first spoke with Jive, apparently she was saying 'Cooee, I'm here!', which was a first for her communications with horses. She told Cheryl that she knew she was overly sensitive, a little neurotic and a 'bit of a pain in the ar**' (her words!), especially when she's in season.

Cheryl told me that there were no real issues with Jive, as long as she is treated with kindness and respect. She is definitely still a little pedantic, especially if she feels she has not been asked 'correctly', in the way that she wants to be. If she doesn't understand what she's being asked, she's just going to plant her feet and stare blankly at you – this is very accurate! All she bothers about is being treated with care and respect. She's also very fond of Mickey, my other horse, she's the boss, though, despite the fact that he dwarfs her.

Cheryl told me that this little pony is definitely 'in charge' and having seen her with my big horse, this is truly the case. During the reading, Jive apologised for her behaviour – she was being affected by her season and wanted me to know that this is not how she generally behaved (we had not owned her for very long at the time of the reading). She definitely felt neurotic and wasn't able to process her feelings. (I think most women can relate to this at certain times of the month!)

Jive thanked me for not letting anyone leap on her back straight away; she appreciated the time to settle in before she started her riding career. She was very happy to receive individual attention, she had come from a large herd and hadn't been used to having her own person. She loves to have a job and is happiest when she's busy. She told Cheryl that she doesn't like lead rein work, she will do it but she's better when she is trusted to do her job, so my daughter will have to get much more practice in.

I was ecstatic to hear that she really likes my daughter, even though she doesn't like all children. Jive appreciates that my little one is kind and polite, which is how she wanted to be treated. Jive enjoys the work that my girl is doing with her – even just handling, grooming and leading around the field. Cheryl picked up that she was tight in her off-shoulder due to the lead reining she had previously done, and asked if we could work on the other side to give her a bit of a break.

I wanted Cheryl to tell Jive that I was sorry I hadn't really spent enough time with her. Both she and my other horse were being looked after, but my mental health was at an all-time low when she first arrived, and I didn't feel I had given her as much as she deserved. Jive's response was 'Why apologise? Not to worry, it can't be helped,' which made me feel infinitely better. Of course, horses are sensitive creatures, and they understand that some days are better than others. It was very reassuring to hear that she didn't mind that I hadn't spent as much time with her as I wanted to.

I asked what her problem was with fly spray, and Jive replied that she has sensitive skin. Thankfully, Cheryl recommended some essential oils that are kinder to the skin, which we now use instead, with much better results. She also really hated fly masks, which I was told is because she doesn't get enough air through them. During Cheryl's remote health check, she told me that Jive's back lower-right-side teeth were a little sharp. I had the dentist booked shortly after for a general check, and they confirmed this.

Her feet were another thing that Cheryl picked up on; they have now been properly dealt with by my farrier and are looking much better. Cheryl also told me that her right eye and the tip of her left ear were crusty – this was indeed true, but the issue came and went without any problems.

Jive remains a cheeky, sassy pony with attitude, but she has a heart of gold and is not dangerous. I don't think she would ever kick or bite or be aggressive, and she loves me and my daughter. I'm very much looking forward to watching their relationship develop over time, and I feel confident that Cheryl will be able to iron out any small problems we may have in the future.

I'm so happy that Cheryl is around, and that she has such an amazing gift, which can really help the relationship between horses and their people. I'm still so blown away by how much knowledge she can have about a horse without even meeting them.

Athena and Enyo – Connie Colfox

I start and retrain horses so have up to forty at my home at any one time. Cheryl has read so many of my horses that it is honestly very difficult to remember individual cases, but I do know that in every single case her reading was spot-on. We work together around four times a year – Cheryl comes to the yard, and we work through the horses one by one. I find this incredibly helpful in getting them started or retrained as I can understand their individual selves better and tailor my workings to them.

A few of the horses that Cheryl's 'read' for me have stuck in my mind, so I'll just go through a few of them. Cheryl first came to talk to my daughter's pony who'd had a complicated background and was not going on very well. I can't remember the ins and outs of the reading (as I said, I have had a lot!), but it was obvious Cheryl was the real deal, so for my birthday I asked Cheryl to come to the yard for the morning and we just went from horse to horse, and she read them.

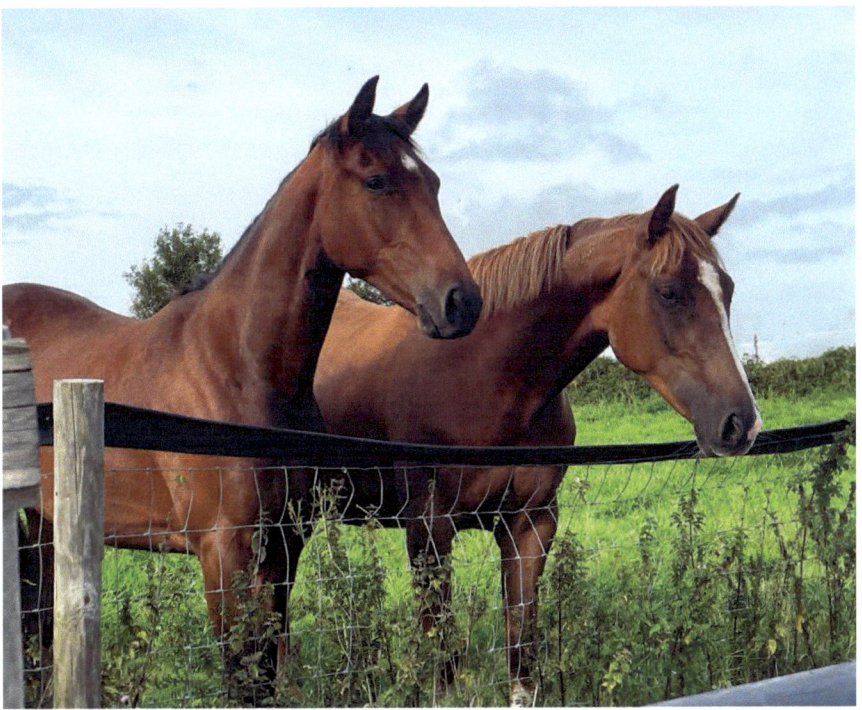

Enyo and Athena. (Connie Colfox)

On that occasion, I had a horse who was clearly not enjoying his training. He hadn't ever done anything bad, but it was very obvious to me that he didn't like being ridden, just by his demeanour. She looked across at him and straight away said that he didn't want to go to his next yard. I didn't really believe this, as the next yard he was going to belonged to a good friend, who'd had a lot of young horses from me and she was a very kind trainer. I also thought, 'Well, how on Earth can he know where he is going?' Cheryl told me this was because the girl had come and ridden him with us, which was true, but not something that Cheryl knew at that point. I still thought this was nonsense, as I knew my friend would do a great job.

The horse went to my friend, and I was with them one day doing cross-country schooling. We were doing the water jump. They both seemed to be doing well and he walked sweetly through the water the first time. Then, on the second time, he went into the water, still looking very sweet – then stopped and absolutely *buried* her. I'd not seen a horse buck so furiously in a very long time. Amazingly she stayed on for quite a while, but then she did, unsurprisingly, fall off. We'd had him at our yard for quite a while and he'd only had one buck in that time, and certainly not as premeditated and violent as the one in front of me. Was this just a coincidence or was he telling me something, because I had been there when Cheryl told me that he didn't want to go to the next yard?

Another interesting case features two of my homebred fillies – Enyo and Athena, two and three years old respectively, who are full sisters. Now, when Cheryl comes to my yard, she barely even looks at the horses – she will ask their names, then pretty much turn her back on them – for me, this adds to the authenticity as it shows that she's not sneakily working anything out about them based on their bodies, their gaits or visible behaviours.

Cheryl told me that Enyo was very keen on being with people, that she had issues with personal space, but that she was a sensible horse and had a very grounded energy. Athena, I was told, was not so confident. She was a watcher and preferred not to participate. She wants to do well, but she's slow to join in. I can't tell you how accurate that was!

I had worked these little fillies a few days before, loose jumping (over a very tiny jump, in case anyone's worried that I'm abusing my youngsters!) because someone was interested in taking on Enyo. They were in the school together for the first time ever, displaying their individual personalities. Enyo took to it like a duck to water; taking everything in her stride and leading confidently over the jump with her ears pricked as if she'd been doing it all her life. Athena, despite being older and a full sister to Enyo, was not *nearly* so confident in the school and was always trailing behind Enyo, not willing to go out and face the world herself.

In the field with Enyo and Athena was Aries – the half-brother to the two fillies. Aries had had some foot problems and had to have remedial foot treatment. After being seen by one of the top vets in the country at the time, who couldn't find anything wrong, Cheryl, after meeting Aries, could feel his string halt. After another meeting with the vet with this information, it was suddenly obvious.

I have another Cheryl experience with a pair of full sisters – Sophie and Ginny. These girls look identical, to the point that I have been known to tack the wrong one up! Cheryl told me that Ginny is not lazy, but that she does the 'minimum required' and that she likes to conserve her energy. She said that she likes to 'babysit the neurotic ones', which was exactly what we had been using her for, despite the fact that she was only four! Ginny wants to have a foal and she would be a good mother – she takes everything in her stride and is generally very easy. She's definitely more whoa than go, and I always feel safe with her. Cheryl told me about her gut problems – Ginny had had a terrible bout of colic and we'd nearly lost her. I was recommended some really useful bits and bobs to help her gut heal. Again, I hadn't told Cheryl anything about the colic or the gut problems prior to the reading.

Sophie is a completely different kettle of fish. She's a much sharper horse, who says that she feels 'a bit let down'. Interestingly, I feel the same about her! Her mother was one of my favourite horses in the world, and I bred from her for this reason, but I didn't feel that Sophie had really lived up to her breeding. Maybe she was picking up on me feeling let down? Cheryl told me that Sophie goes out of her way to be awkward, that she will *not* be rushed, and that you can't cut corners. This is Sophie to a tee, and we have had to take a lot of extra care with her training. She's now going really well with the extra attention and care I take with her and she is getting past her anxieties.

One more horse I can tell you about came from a top, top competition home (I can't honestly say much more, sorry if this sounds like a spy novel!) and who was on his way to jump in the Olympics. I had never ridden a horse that felt so unbalanced – it felt as though he would fall over if I let go of the reins. He went back to his owner and I thought that he was going to be checked out, but it turns out he hadn't been. He had a problem with his reining back when he returned to me a year later, and he told Cheryl that he had completely lost his joy in life. When we were in the school, his eyes looked completely dead. He also had a lot of health problems, from hindgut to tightness in the legs and back. He wanted to stay with me and stated that I needed to 'fight his corner'. I will always feel bad that I didn't make quite enough fuss about getting him more looked at – it turned out that he had no less than seven kissing spines. I wish I had stamped my foot a lot more about him.

These are a tiny fraction of the horses at my yard that Cheryl has communicated with; I have to stop there, or we'll be here all week.

Whenever I say to Cheryl, I'm not sure she's right about something (I'm never worried about saying that to Cheryl, as she hasn't got an ego), a few days or even months later the horse will show me that I was wrong and Cheryl was right.

I have always believed there is more to a horse than is obvious, and that they have thoughts and feelings and are advanced beings. As a horse trainer I think it's really important to remember this, and I want to do my best for the horses. Having Cheryl come to the yard amazes me every time. I just love it. It's my favourite day. I love to go around and hear what is going on inside their heads. I also think it has made me more intuitive to them and helped me as a trainer to look outside the box and be more sensitive to their needs – and yes, this helps me get better results, too.

Florian and Hawk – Jilly Sowdon

Florian is a lovely cob cross who I bred myself from two ponies, neither of whom were over 14hh. Florian was intended to be my forever riding horse, but he has matured into a mountain of 16.2hh, and as I am only 5ft 4in and in my sixties, I was a little concerned as to what would happen when he was old enough to ride. My daughter had her pony read by Cheryl, with amazing results, so I decided to see what my horses would say. Well, in my old age and cynicism, I thought 'Oh yes, I have heard of people who advertise their magical skills, charge a lot and say no more than an owner or keeper can discern for themselves by just tuning into their horse.' Goodness, I was proved wrong!

Cheryl spoke to Florian and described him as a 'bit of a Kevin the Teenager', which is very accurate! He has since been started and was true to Cheryl's suggestion that he would never canter, he is something of an ambler.

I had recently bought a little pony with an extraordinary personality, Hawk, because it was clear that Florian was too much horse for me! I fell in love with Hawk on my first visit and he seemingly did so with me, but once he was home with my other horses, he appeared so vastly changed and distant, that I couldn't work it out. It wasn't just the usual 'let them

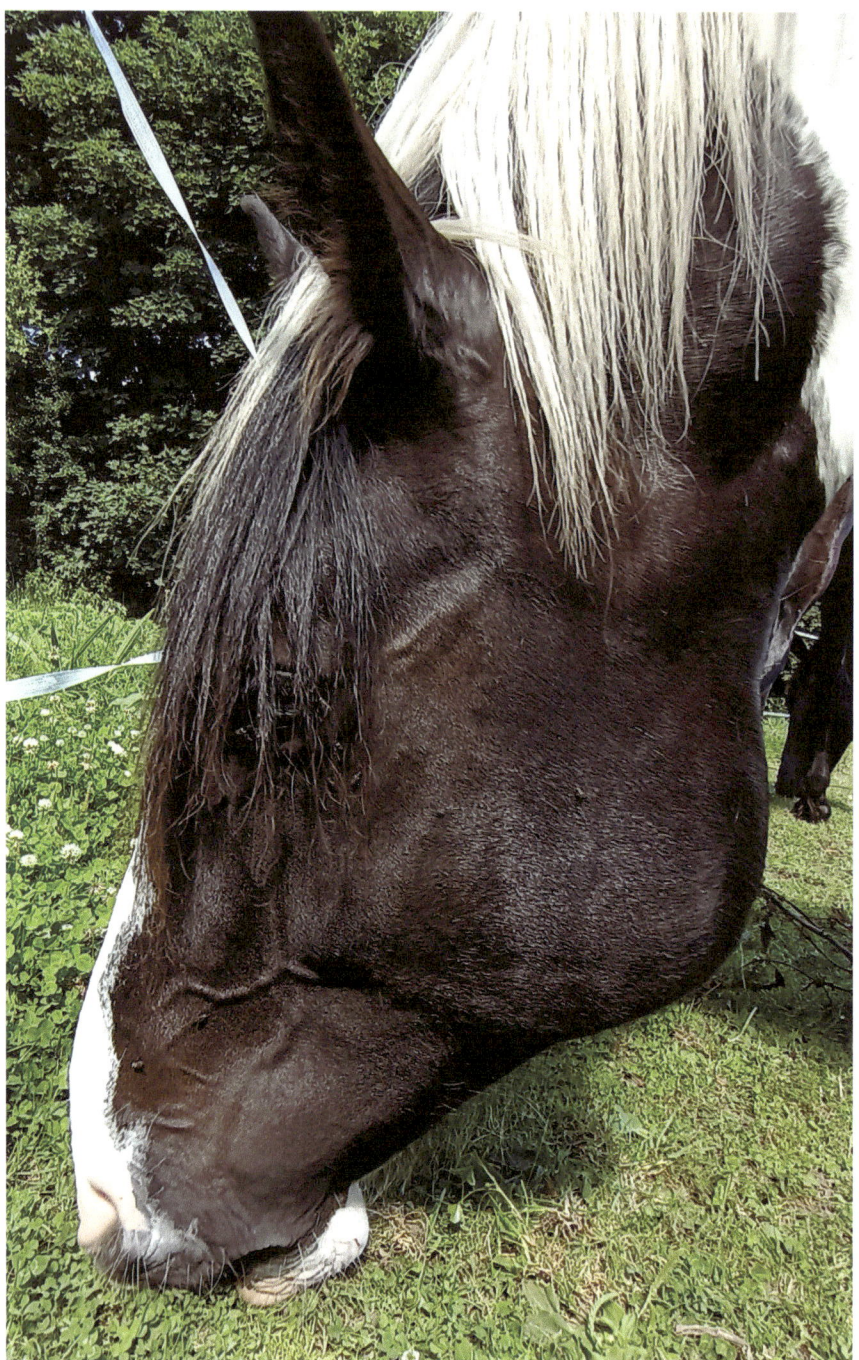

Florian. (Jilly Sowdon)

settle in' kind of issue that one has with a new horse, it was as if I had completely misread him, and I felt lost. Having heard the amazing feedback of my daughter's reading from Cheryl I thought I would contact her, still not really believing that she could help me and the pony, but my goodness, she cleared so many small points for us both, it was very obvious that she was the real deal, the genuine horse talker.

Hawk told Cheryl that he was very happy to be with me and was really looking forward to 'taking me up the hill and across the top', but would I please take lots of time with him and take it slowly. Cheryl pointed out he had a left-side-tooth issue, which I had half-wondered about as he seemed a bit mouthy on that side. He said to her that please would I not sedate him when the dentist came, which I won't!

There were many small chats about the others in the field, which helped tremendously as I hadn't previously thought of how each horse sees their position and job in the herd. I had only checked that they were comfortable and content, and missed the small tensions, which when we know we can talk to the horse, explain that we know how they feel and that we understand them. Yes, really!

Cheryl told me that to just tell them, in an ordinary conversational way, would help both the horse and owner to clear small problems and she is right. Now, every day when there is something that is going to happen, I tell them all and sometimes sit with one individually as they munch hay or I give them a groom, and I can feel them shift in a way that is difficult to describe.

I know this works by the way things are when I forget to talk, like the day Florian came back from being started. I was so focused on making sure that he would be okay to come out for a walk on his own with me, that I did not tell all the others that he was going out and that they would be okay on their hay for half an hour or so, and that he *would* be coming back. This caused a flurry of neighing, some busting through electric tape and a general feeling of anxiety and stress.

It is so rarely the horse's fault when things are a bit rubbish in field or stable; it is 99 per cent of the time, our misreading or lack of comprehension of the horse. We forget to treat them as cognitive beings, when they so truly are. This is the magic that Cheryl helped me to see. I am truly grateful for her clarity and insight.

Rafi – Serena Bower

Rafi is a cob cross – possibly crossed with a shire, although we don't really know! He is twelve and built like a beautiful tank.

I first asked for Cheryl's advice because I noticed that he wasn't moving as well as he usually does and seemed very

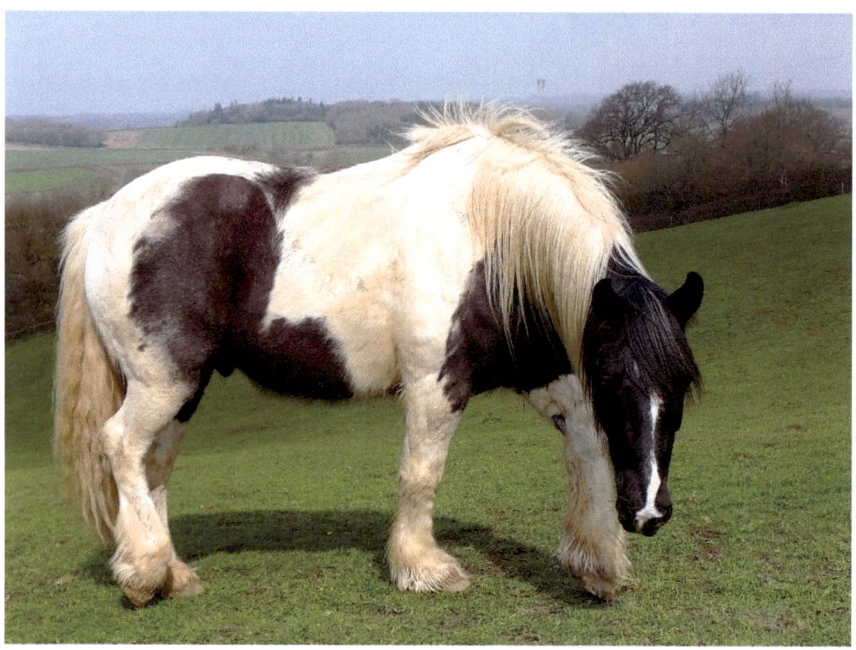

Rafi. (Serena Bower)

sore through his lower back. I am an equine McTimoney chiropractor, but even all my tricks weren't working to help him feel more comfortable consistently – he would release, but then the problem would come back again very quickly. I contacted a physio who was a specialist nerve releaser, and an osteopath but nothing worked. You know your own horse, and I just knew that all was not right with Rafi – despite the fact that he didn't seem too bad. I was also concerned that he might have a problem with his guts, and wanted some insights on what was going on with my boy.

On our phone call, Cheryl told me that usually she has a back-and-forth conversation with a horse, but that Rafi didn't even draw breath! He just wanted to get it all off his chest because he knew that I was worried about him. He mentioned a very specific date to Cheryl – June, two years ago – and said that I was not there. I had been in Portugal at that time, so this was spot-on. He said that he'd been playing around in the field with one of his companions when he slipped and fell, and it had affected his sacroiliac joint. No one picked it up at the time. Fast-forward to the following spring, I was bringing him back into work and doing some lungeing, when he slipped and fell, coming down on the off-fore – this exacerbated the problem even further.

It has been very helpful to me to know what Rafi's problem is, as I can tailor my treatments specifically for that area, in the hope of making him more comfortable. I did chuckle during the reading, as apparently, he told Cheryl to tell me there is nothing wrong with his eyesight; he can be clumsy and I often ask him if he can see! I also learned that his guts were fine, so that was a weight off my mind. I heard that he was happy with his saddle and bridle, and that he likes the way I ride – I try to guide him using my seat and voice, which he is very responsive to.

Interestingly, I have a lot of clients locally and I would say that at least 50 per cent of them have had Cheryl read their horses, and all have nothing but good things to say about her – as do I.

Jessie Joop – Jessica Longstaffe

This is Jessie Joop's story and it's probably very different to others you may have read, with an ending that I wish was different, but it doesn't change the fact Cheryl helped us more than I could ask with Jessie.

My mum and I bought Jessie in January 2021, a 15.2hh Irish sports horse cross cob. She was, on paper, my type to an absolute tee. A beautiful chunky sporty cob! We were sold Jessie as a mother–daughter share, who had been there done that, was not spooky and one who would give confidence. My mum had been out of the saddle for years, so it was really important to both of us for her to have a safe ride. Jessie was fabulous on her trial, but in hindsight she was definitely doped or starved to reduce her energy levels – something the notorious dealer was known for, but obviously we didn't know this at the time.

Jessie started off great; the first few days she was perfect, but that soon began to change. She became very unpredictable, one minute she was calm and relaxed, the next she was scared of everything and everyone. This went on for weeks and then months. It resulted in some major falls for my mum and others around us, one of which ended up with Mum having a lengthy stay in hospital with broken ribs, a punctured lung and damage to her kidney. The strange part was I never had an explosion from Jessie, we had so much fun, but I could see the damage she had done to others, which frightened me. However, we were determined to keep trying.

Case Studies

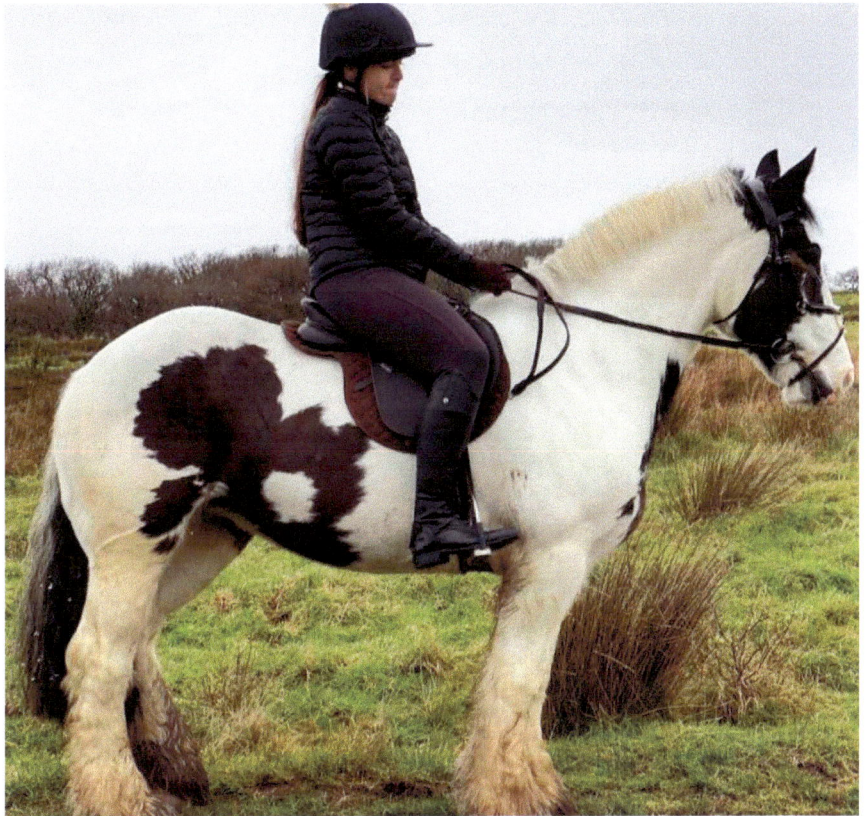

Jessie Joop. (Jessica Longstaff)

We had every professional you could think of the vet, physio, farrier and dentist. There was absolutely no set trigger for Jessie's explosions and they were exactly that. Blind bolting, throwing every shape possible just to get herself away from the situation. Each time she had her moments, she would dismount her rider and then you'd find her with her head down, shaking and with the most kind-but-sorry look in her eyes. I knew that this wasn't coming from a place of malice, Jessie had the kindest soul. I bonded with her so much, unfortunately but understandably, though, my mum struggled to trust and bond with her after several serious falls.

We were told about Cheryl through a friend who had used her before. I admit I was sceptical but at this point we had spent thousands, suffered heartbreak, and with so much faith lost it was worth trying. Cheryl came out, and still to this day I can't quite explain the feeling I had when she walked into our barn and Jessie's reaction. With anyone else Jessie would have either become very fidgety and flighty, or completely shied away. But not with Cheryl. Jessie stood there calm and happy while Cheryl began to communicate with her, and within minutes told us she was 'sorry for the stag incident'; this was the accident that Jessie and Mum had, which put Mum into hospital for the long stay. Immediately we knew Cheryl was absolutely spot-on as we hadn't told her any details about the accident, and we were hooked.

We were told about a previous cart accident; that the personalities of me and my mum balanced each other out for Jessie, and she liked it. Also, that no matter what bit she had in her mouth it wouldn't stop her. There was so much information gained that we needed to hear. The part that hit me most, and still gets me, was that Jessie told us she knew there was a chance she wouldn't be with us forever and she may not be the horse for us, but she was so grateful that we were trying harder than anyone had before.

Cheryl helped us so much; we started groundwork and our bond grew even stronger. We sent Jessie to Connie Colfox, who was recommended by Cheryl, and the difference in Jessie at her yard was unbelievable – I couldn't believe it. Unfortunately, I believe there was a lot of trauma at our yard that may have stuck with Jessie, so when she came home things soon got back to normal for us.

We came to the heartbreaking decision to sell Jessie; this was the hardest thing I have ever agreed to do. It breaks my heart every day. Jessie was sold as a broodmare and we strongly stated she was not to be ridden; unfortunately this didn't happen. She was picked up by a seemingly lovely gentleman who bred cobs, but sadly and disgustingly he was working undercover for a dealer, who then sold Jessie on in the same way she was sold to us. I longed for the chance to get Jessie back, but I couldn't bring myself to search for her because the guilt was eating me alive. I couldn't ride, I couldn't be around horses and I'm sure everyone around me was fed up with me talking about Jessie. I couldn't explain the bond we had and the kindness I saw in her, but I knew Cheryl would understand.

We got a lovely new mare for my mum who was absolutely perfect and I couldn't wish for a better pony for her. However, I couldn't bond with her and still to this day I can't. It's because she isn't Jessie. I decided to get Cheryl out for the new mare Beau, as I knew she could help us and, deep down, I was hoping she could tell me something about Jessie. And incredibly, but not surprisingly, she did. As soon as Cheryl arrived, I think it was clear how much my mum was in love with Beau, but I was not. Then I asked about Jessie, and Cheryl requested a picture of her eye. I found one and Cheryl, amazingly, was able to give me a rough location of North Yorkshire or the Lincolnshire area. I took a few days to think about it. Then I went on to Find My Horse UK and posted Jessie's photos and details. Within minutes I discovered that Jessie was at a sales livery in Lincolnshire, but a week before had been at a riding school in North Yorkshire. I was honestly amazed and so happy. Sadly, I explained everything to the new owners and offered to buy her, but they were asking thousands, which I didn't have.

I found Jessie five more times since; sadly, I have never been able to afford to buy her back. There's not a day goes by that

I don't think of my sweet Jessie Joop. I saw Cheryl earlier this year by sheer chance, and again plucked up the courage to talk about Jessie. Cheryl told me something that I hold with me every day; one day Jessie will be back with me and that our story isn't over. Out of everybody I contacted during Jessie's journey, Cheryl was by far the most rewarding, the most amazing and the most helpful. I cannot thank her enough.

I still think about Jessie every day, but I have hope and faith in Cheryl's words that one day I will have our Jessie back home.

Murphy – Gail North

Murphy's a chestnut Irish sports horse, he's fifteen years old and 16.3hh. I bought him as a gangly seven-year-old and he's now finally grown into his legs!

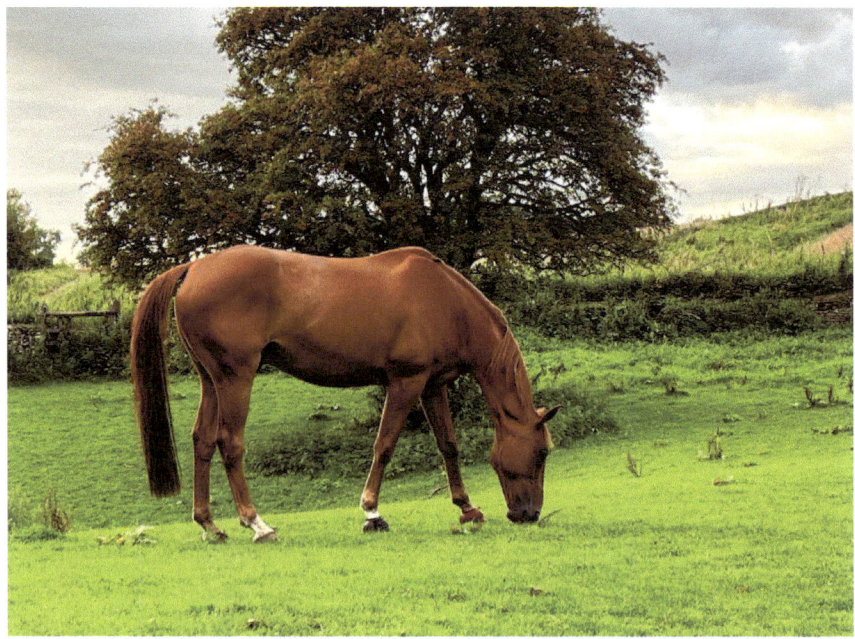

Murphy. (Gail North)

I can't remember the reason I first contacted Cheryl over seven years ago – pure curiosity, I think – she'd been recommended by a highly cynical friend, so I thought 'Why not?' A standout comment from one of the early calls was along the lines of 'he holds his head higher than you'd like' – in truth he was a little like a ginger giraffe, and the 'correct' muscles in his neck were highly underdeveloped and he braced through his under neck. She also mentioned he travelled well and almost went to sleep while doing so. Murphy at the time was quite a stressful, spooky horse, but one of the things he did incredibly calmly was load and travel.

As each session went on and he became more comfortable in himself, his cheeky personality came out. I had one reading about the time he has been diagnosed with arthritis and treated for ulcers. Apparently, he

'didn't know what all the fuss was about'. He said he hoped 'that man' wouldn't be coming back, which, given that he had a challenging scope recently I thought he meant the vet. In hindsight I suspect he meant the farrier who refused to shoe Murphy as he said he was dangerous to shoe. He's now an absolute dream to shoe, or do anything with his feet, and I frequently receive comments on how good he is.

I had been going through a particularly stressful time and his behaviour, especially when ridden, was getting worse. I'd had a couple of people mention that I should get rid of him, of which there was no chance, but I was pretty sure that how I was feeling was contributing to how he was.

'Tell her to just stop and do nothing with me for a while,' was a little thing I could do for him he said. Around the same time as this, we started the academic art of riding, which at times to observers may have looked like we were standing and doing nothing. However, with this approach,

Murphy started to slowly change and relax far more, and our relationship improved no end. In the first session with Cheryl after starting this, I remember her saying he really enjoyed it, and for me to just picture what I wanted and he would 'give it a go'.

At our next session, I remember Cheryl saying excitedly how amazingly our relationship had shifted; something had happened about six or eight months ago that had changed us both, that he was far more considerate of me and would – despite sometimes finding it difficult – not overreact and apologised for not being there for me when I needed him.

In that time, we'd found a different trainer who focused a lot on energy while working with horses and had helped me work through how I was turning up for him. It was amazing to hear Murphy (via Cheryl) echo how I felt things were going. She could still feel a few niggles physically, and hacking was a really stressful experience, but she said to keep working how we were and apply what we had learned in the school while out and about, and it would come.

Our most recent couple of sessions continued to build on this, and Cheryl could feel how much stronger and more balanced he was and explained why he kept standing in front of the mirror in the school: 'He's showing you how square he is in front now, he's very pleased with it.'

We'd also really struggled to keep shoes on through the summer, and I was in the paddock looking for another lost shoe and I thought to myself 'Please show me where you lost it!' At that point one of his field mates squealed and cantered off, I went to where he had been standing, followed some hoof marks and found a shoe. Unsure if it was a coincidence or not, I asked again, at which point he moved to another part of the field and kept nodding. Feeling slightly silly I ignored him, then went across and managed to move him out the way and there was another shoe. When I asked Cheryl about the shoe, she said Murphy was pleased as he had been pointing it out to me.

Our most recent session was after he'd had his shoes off, it was a quick catch-up to confirm he was feeling better after giving him some milk thistle. Not only was his liver feeling better, but Cheryl said, 'He says he's lovely, and I can feel he's moving smoother and standing different.' In between the sessions I'd had his shoes removed and we were beginning the transition to barefoot. A friend of mine who is an equine podiatrist gave his feet a look over and helped me measure for boots and kept saying how lovely he was, and we were all quite surprised how he was moving more freely without his shoes. He was confirming and quite happy about being called 'lovely'.

One of the standout themes of each of our sessions is Cheryl frequently saying, 'You'll know, he'll tell you,' which has helped enormously on our journey. At first his communication could be quite loud and explosive, now it's far more quiet and subtle, though clearer, and the change in him has been unbelievable. Many of the physical things Cheryl has noted have been confirmed by the farrier/chiropractor/vet, though the main thing is that the confirmation of what I feel he has been trying to say – particularly in the past couple of years – has been the same as what he's said to Cheryl. She has played a huge part in this improved relationship. I love our three-way chats and feel it has really helped in our understanding of each other, and our communication overall. Although it's all still a work in progress, that spooky ginger lunatic is becoming a distant memory. He's now one of the most relaxed horses in the yard, and Cheryl's gift has had a huge part in supporting that and bringing out the best of my Murphy.

Jasper and Hendrik – Chloe Holland

I keep a large mixed herd of horses on a track system that my husband and I designed and built, and I also take in liveries. I often get Cheryl out to talk to the whole herd, whether they are mine or not, as this can really help with working out the herd dynamic of who's happy with whom, what's working for each horse and, of course, any health issues that they may have. These are just a couple of the standout stories I have from Cheryl's visits.

Jasper is my cob, who I bought to bring back my confidence after a couple of bad accidents – he's a ten-year-old 'steady

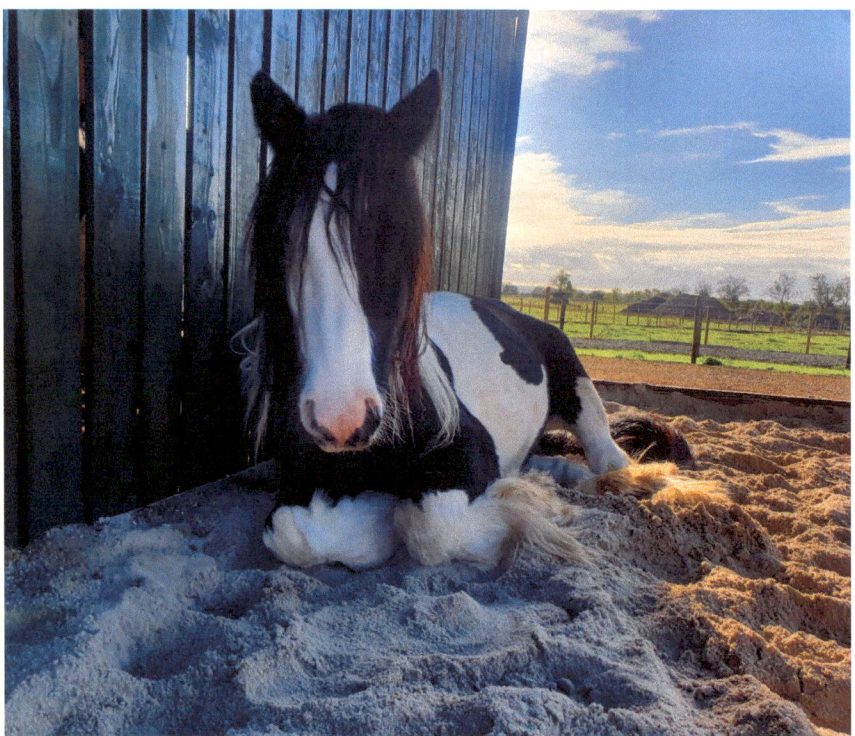

Jasper. (Chloe Holland)

Neddy' type. He's pretty calm, collected and sure of his place in the herd, and he's my main riding horse. I took him to a cross-country clinic, but he hadn't really had enough preparation and training, and it blew his mind! I had to get my instructor to ride him, as he just turned into a fireball and I didn't want to lose my nerve all over again. It made me cry – it wasn't pretty! He was like that the whole session; he was clearly struggling with what he was being asked to do and even with my instructor on board he carried on losing the plot (she had to conduct the lesson from on board my bucking bronco, which obviously wasn't ideal!).

A couple of days later, Cheryl arrived to read the herd. Jasper is usually the first one to come and talk to her; he actually seeks her out. Well, on this particular day he was nowhere to be seen – then we spotted him, right at the top of the track, just staring down, all on his own. I wasn't sure if Cheryl could talk to him over the 15m between us, but she checked in. She looked at me and said, 'He's embarrassed. He doesn't want to come down.' I thought that was a bit odd, so I asked her to ask him why. She went quiet, then said, 'He's embarrassed about your last ride.' Suddenly I remembered that our last ride had been that awful day at the cross-country clinic. Poor Jasper felt very silly about it. We let him know that it was okay and that it wasn't a problem, but I felt bad for the poor boy.

When I first got Jasper, he told Cheryl that he was happy to do the job of being my next horse, but that I must stop calling him a 'doughnut'. I used to call him this all the time if he was doing anything silly, as an alternative to swearing! I have stopped doing this and surprise, surprise, he does seem much happier.

Hendrik is my big, beautiful Friesian boy, who often wanders around behind me as I'm doing jobs, and who I often talk to.

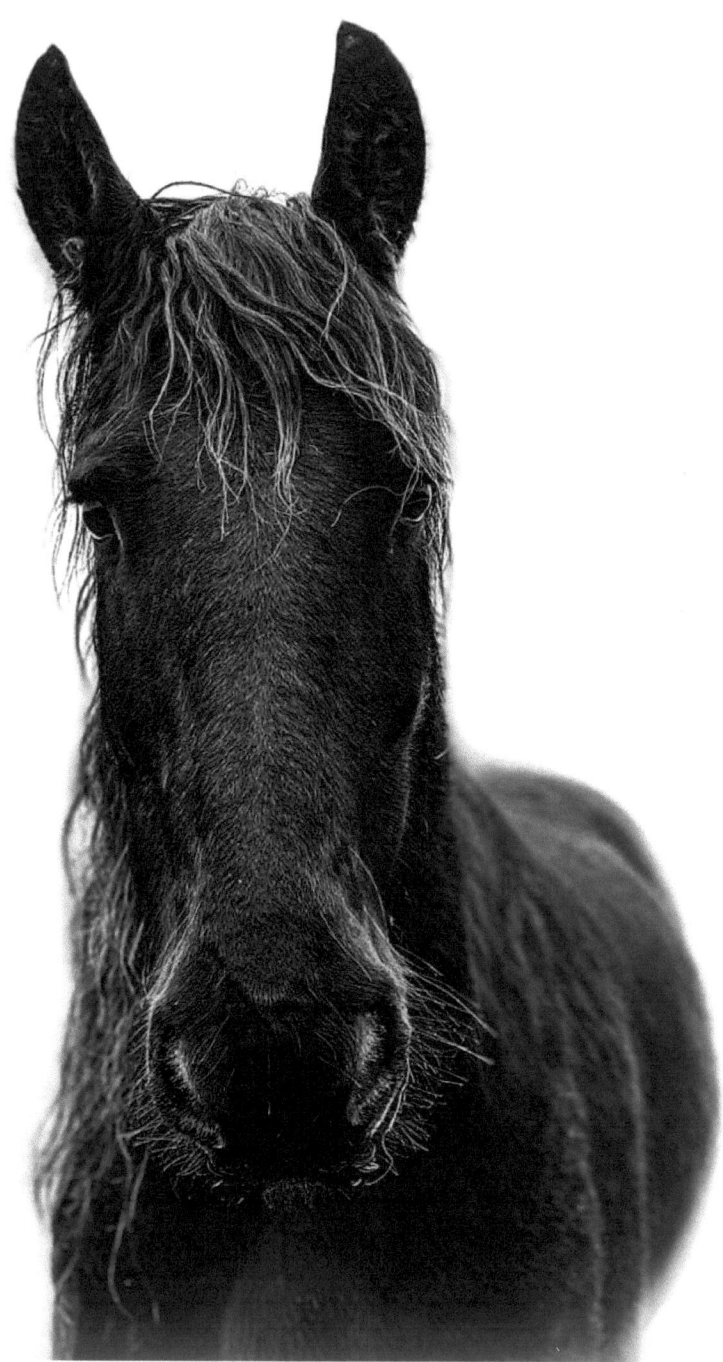

Hendrik. (Chloe Holland)

As I was designing the new track system, I had been wondering what to do at the top end, where it wasn't particularly safe. I'd planned for the top half to be stone and the bottom half to be sand. I had drawn the plans, but not told anyone about it – apart from Hendrik. I'd always assumed that horses respond to the tone of voice more than the actual words we use, but I found out that this is not the case.

During one of Cheryl's visits, Hendrik came over for a chat. Cheryl told me that Hendrik approved of my new plans for the track. I tried to not give too much away to Cheryl – not because I don't trust her, but obviously it could be a generic thing to say, and I asked her what he meant by that. She described everything that I had told Hendrik, and even drew a little rough picture of it on the barn floor! I found that a little creepy, but absolutely spot-on, as always.

12

PEOPLE HEARING WITHOUT LISTENING

I hope you don't mind the song quote, but it just seemed apt. We all want to be the best people for our horses that we can be – and we want them to be their best selves, too. So, how can you get on with hearing your own horse more, understanding their needs and making the very best of your partnership, without necessarily enlisting the help of an equine communicator?

There are a good few things you can do to develop a deeper communication with your horse – and none of these things will mean radically changing the way you do things, or investing in expensive equipment, or turning your horse into a pampered diva who never has to do the things you want. Sometimes it is just about opening your mind a little.

Well, the phrase 'trust your gut' is wildly overused, but in this case it is very fitting. Listening to those little voices in your head is one of the things, in this day and age, that we need to be doing more and more. Listening to your intuition is very underrated. Horses have a very highly tuned intuition – possibly because they were originally prey animals, and ignoring a niggling feeling could mean the difference between life and death. One thing that

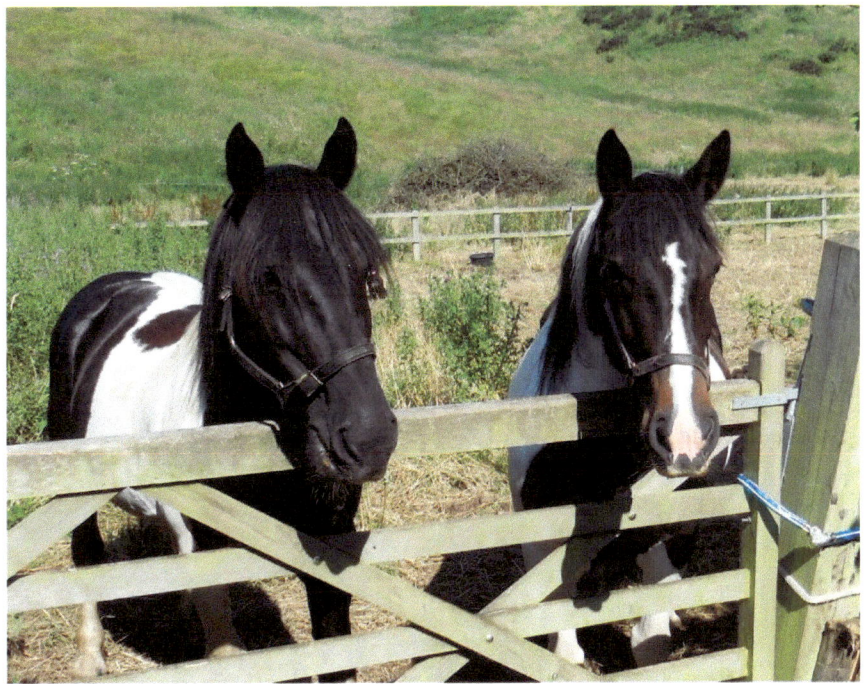

They're always ready to listen. (Jilly Sowdon)

I regularly say to clients is, I don't care how many years someone has worked with horses or how many letters they have after their name, if it doesn't sit right in your gut, *never* ignore it, that is your horse shouting at you.

Listen to your horse, pay attention to those niggling feelings. If it doesn't feel like the right day to ride, or your horse is definitely 'off' while you're loading to go on that pleasure ride, then do yourselves a favour, take a deep breath and realise that this is not the be all and end all. We all need a duvet day once in a while and your horse is no different. If you push them too hard when they're just not feeling it, chances are you might end up on the deck.

Talk to your horse; tell them what's going on, even if you feel stupid. Luckily *all* animals are telepathic, so you can do this quietly in your head. Mind you, that does mean that they hear you just as effectively if you are next to them, at your coffee table at home, or sitting sipping a cocktail on a faraway beach, so mind what you say! Horses are incredibly intelligent animals; they can recognise faces, they know members of their herd even when they haven't seen them for years, and yes, they *do* understand what you are saying to them.

Taking the time to set your intentions, even if that is just telling them 'we are going for a little wander around the lanes today', will have a big impact on how they do. If they know what to expect, things will go much better. Think of it as the same way that you would explain to your child that 'Yes, it *is* school today.' Treat your horse with at least the same amount of love, compassion and respect as you would your children (after all, for many of us these enormous creatures *are* our family).

Ask for permission. You don't have to wait for them to consider a reply, especially if it is for something that you know is non-negotiable, but making sure you take their feelings into account is important. It's the same way that you might ask a toddler, 'I'm going to change your nappy now, is that okay?' You know it's going to happen, they know it's going to happen, you know that even if they say no, you're still going to do it, because it's essential for them – but it's just good manners to ask. Horses appreciate this.

Appreciate them. We all know what it's like to go through the day-to-day and feel like no one acknowledges you, let alone thanks you. As much as you do, your horse deserves to know when they've done a clever thing that they haven't managed to do before, or when they've tried their hearts out for you. Always say 'thank you'.

They are living creatures, not machines; they have thoughts and opinions and desires and wishes just like us. It can be easy to think that horses are just 'stop/start' creatures but, let's face it, if you have horses then you *know* this isn't the case. The more we know them, spend time with them, work with them, and learn and grow with them, the more we realise that horses really are special creatures.

Treat them like the sentient beings they are, tell them you understand them and want to do the best for them. Often, even just telling them that you *are* listening to them can stop a tantrum in its tracks. Who in the world doesn't want to hear that their feelings are valid, and that they are cared about?

Spend time just sitting and being – not riding, grooming or working – just sitting in the field, watching and being part of the herd. This is especially important with very nervous horses, or those who have suffered trauma and associate people with pain or discomfort. Sitting in the stable or the field, just pottering about and letting them know you are there, will do wonders for your relationship. I know it's not always easy to find the time, but take a flask of tea, even a good book or a phone to fiddle about on and let your horses feel your presence.

Talking and listening to your horse doesn't have to be something you do in secret or feel silly about, just remember that they are beings, too, and they deserve love, respect, and appreciation as much as you do. If you haven't done so before, give it a try – just chat to them about what you're doing, ask them how they are, tell them how much you love them. I promise you; it *will* make a difference.

13

FREQUENTLY ASKED QUESTIONS

1) **When was the first time you knew that you could talk to horses?**
   I guess I had always been doing it, but the first time that made me sit up and take notice was when Ranger got caught in barbed wire, and I just *knew* that he needed me. I always had an affinity for 'difficult' horses because of him, and maybe for this reason I am very easily able to tap into the troubled ones.

2) **Can you talk to other animals?**
   In a word, yes. My business also covers cats and dogs, but I can communicate with every animal I have ever encountered. The most exotic was a beluga whale, named Xavier. This was only a couple of years after I set up my communicating business, and I remember that the resort staff were incredibly surprised when I told them that Xavier, 'Didn't want to go back in with the babies, and that's why he keeps swimming to the centre of the pool.' They had been trying to catch him for months, to put him back with the younger whales – hopefully after I left, they let him stay with the grown-ups where he wanted to be.

Frequently Asked Questions

3) **Can you hear people without them knowing?**
   If I chose to, I could. I don't choose to, because this would be a gross invasion of someone's privacy. Also, I don't want to know what's going on in the deepest, darkest regions of people's minds. It's your business; I have enough of my own, thanks! Never be worried that I'll tap into your mind like I do your horse – your thoughts are safe with you.

4) **Do you hear them as a voice in your head, or is it just like hearing your own thoughts?**
   Generally, it's my own voice. It's just like hearing myself think – but I know for a fact it's not me thinking, because I cannot remember the last time I had a problem with my pasterns, or wanted to complain that my friend was taking all the best hay.

5) **Can you talk to foreign animals?**
   I know I can, because I have spoken to animals who are native to other countries, but there doesn't appear to be any kind of language barrier as the information comes through in English. I would guess that every communicator hears in their own language; it would be interesting to meet up with communicators from other countries and see what their experiences are.

6) **Do they have accents?**
   I have only ever noticed accents on five of the countless horses I have spoken to – maybe they were very strong in their individuality, who knows. There were two with Irish accents, two German, and one that spoke in the broadest West Country accent I have ever heard. I remember this one being very sweet, and so relaxed with his reiki treatment that his owner was genuinely worried he was going to fall over!

7) **Can you feel their pain in your own body?**
Yes. Sometimes it is overwhelming and unbearable, and it is how I am able to be so accurate with pinpointing where the horse is feeling pain, because when I am talking to them or touching them, I feel their pain as if it was my own. I have to be careful if an owner has a physical problem and is too close while I am reading the horse as I have, on occasion, picked up on the owner's problems, too.

8) **How do you walk through a field of horses without being bombarded?**
This is a pretty easy one, I can easily shut out the voices, because I have to consciously 'tune in' when I am communicating with them. Being around horses with whom I am not trying to communicate is easy; I just don't try to communicate with them!

9) **Do you have to consciously choose to listen to them, or can you just do it all the time?**
I consciously choose. I have to be aware of myself, the horse, and in many cases there are specific questions that the owner wants the horse to answer. If I heard them all the time, I imagine it would be very difficult to do my job without feeling like I was in a room with half a dozen people shouting at me all at once.

10) **Is it tiring?**
Honestly, it is utterly exhausting. I love it, don't get me wrong, but it does take a pretty hefty toll, both physically and mentally. I make sure that I have at least half an hour between clients, so that I can have a rest and 'clear' them out of my mind. In the past, I have not been careful with my time and have worked myself to the point of burn-out, but I am trying harder to make sure I get enough breaks and time to recharge myself.

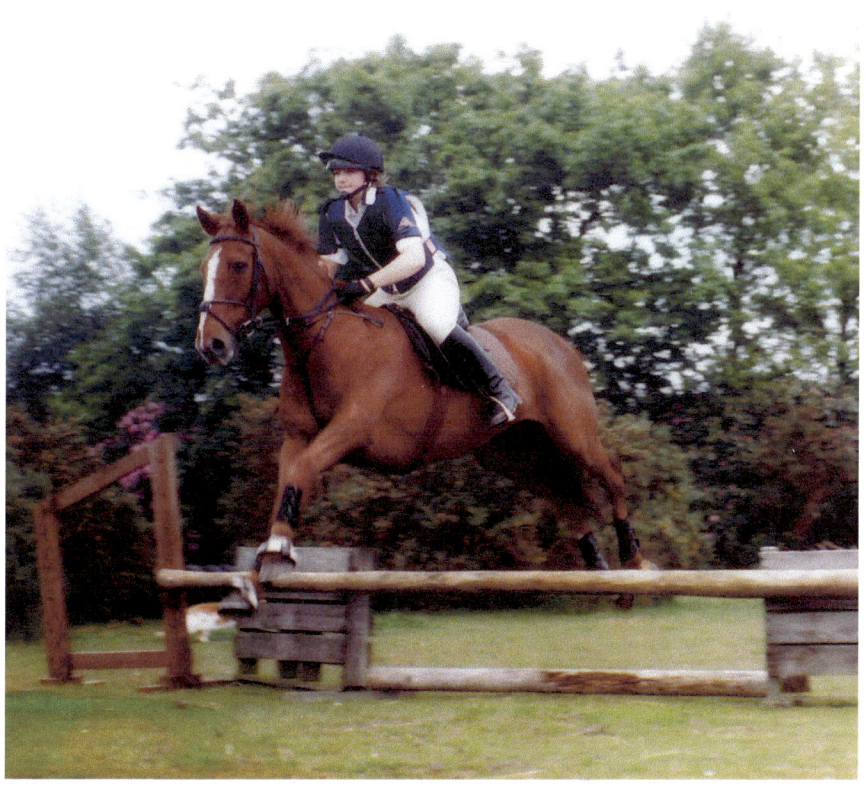

From a young age, Cheryl knew that horses would be central to her life. (George 'Dusty' Miller, BEM, MSM)

ACKNOWLEDGEMENTS

There are a lot of people to be very grateful to, without whom this book would not have seen the light of day.

First and foremost, thank you to Cheryl's wonderful clients who sent in their stories of their experiences with Cheryl, and kindly donated pictures of their beautiful horses. It's been such a pleasure working with you all.

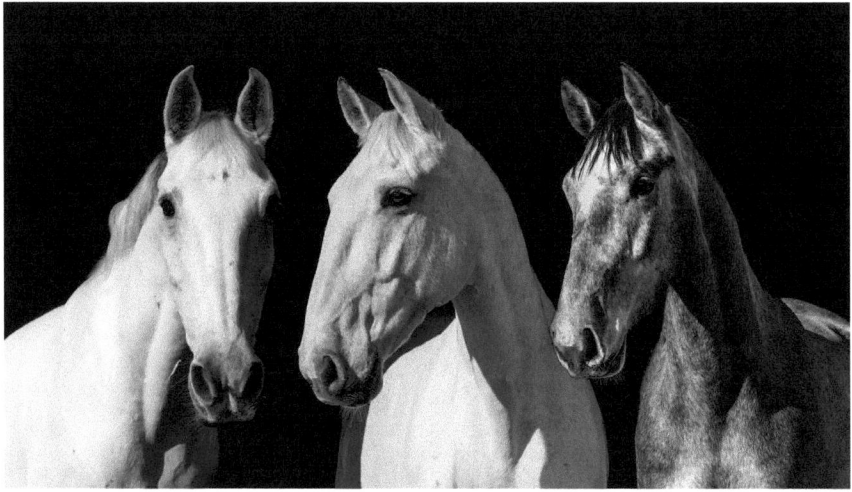

Horses are intelligent enough to understand you, so get chatting! (Katherine Eden Photography)

Acknowledgements

Serena Bower and Lotty Merry, with their invaluable information about how Bowen and McTimoney work.

Anna Curtis of Humble Hooves, for her willingness to share everything she knows about feet (it's a lot!).

The Cornish Ranch Track Livery and Chloe Holland for donating wonderful pictures of track systems.

The fantastic folk at Kenilworth Press who have been supportive, professional and helpful throughout the entire process.

Thank you all so much. We are delighted to bring you this book, and we hope you love reading it as much as we have enjoyed working on it.

INDEX

accommodation 61
aggression 30, 56, 98
antimicrobial 43, 92, 93
arthritis 43, 173

balancers 42
barefoot 57, 59, 61, 117, 135, 175
behaviour 17, 28, 30, 75, 76, 77, 78, 105, 119, 156
behavioural issues 34, 35, 36, 45, 46, 69, 73, 76, 95
blue yarrow 91
body language 15, 16, 118
bodywork 10, 16, 26, 28, 29, 30, 31, 38, 146
bodyworkers 10, 28, 29, 38
Bowen 10, 26, 28, 29, 31, 33, 34, 35, 105, 106, 112, 117, 189

bridle 83, 85, 119, 131, 135, 167

chiropractor 26, 167
cleavers 50
colic 46, 96, 135, 139, 161
communicate 7, 8, 14, 15, 16, 22, 25, 73, 78, 83, 101, 129, 162, 170, 184, 186
communicating 9, 14, 15, 16, 18, 23, 30, 95, 105, 122, 152, 184, 186
communication 15, 16, 29, 30, 34, 140, 156, 175, 180
cow parsley 49
Curtis, Anna 189
cushing's 123

dandelion 49
diet 60, 61
digestion 39, 41, 56, 92

Index

digestive issues 43
digestive system 28, 39, 48, 49

Emmett 35, 36
Emmett points 35, 36
equine communicator 8, 15, 16, 20, 180
essential oil 87, 88, 89, 90, 94, 98, 123, 157
essential oils 87, 89, 93
event fracture 63
exercise 61, 62
extrovert 79

farrier 26, 35, 37, 57, 59, 61, 63, 117, 157, 169, 173, 175
feet 57

garlic 43
GMO ingredients 42
grapefruit 92
gut feelings 39

hawthorn 48
hay 40, 41, 42, 44, 46, 51, 56, 60, 69, 78, 165, 166, 185
hazel 48, 49
hedgerow plants 47, 48, 56
hemlock 49
hooves 28, 44, 57, 58, 59, 60, 61, 62, 63, 89, 96
horse food 41, 42, 108

introvert 79, 117
introverted 79
intuition 180

jasmine 91, 92

kidneys 49

laminitis 40, 43, 46, 48, 50, 57, 61, 70
laminitis 60
lavender 90, 117
liver function 43

massage 31, 32, 33, 37
McCaffrey, Anne 14, 20
McTimoney 31, 36, 37, 98, 167, 189

nervous system 39, 40, 45
nettles 51

obesity 40
oregano 89, 92, 93
osteopath 26, 28, 167

pain 11, 12, 17, 27, 29, 30, 31, 32, 33, 34, 36, 37, 41, 73, 75, 79, 80, 92, 98, 100, 104, 106, 107, 122, 132, 134, 137, 139, 140, 142, 146, 147, 149, 152, 156, 183, 186
peppermint 92

physio 32
physiotherapy 31, 32
poisoning 101

ragwort 70
Ranger 9, 10, 11, 14, 19, 20, 21, 22, 23, 24, 25, 65, 184
red clover 49
reiki 15, 37, 101, 185
rosehip 50
rosemary 91
rotation 71
rug 76, 83, 86, 137, 140

sacroiliac joint 29, 167
saddle 21, 26, 28, 30, 31, 35, 79, 81, 82, 83, 84, 86, 100, 107, 131, 135, 141, 146, 147, 167, 168
saddle fit 26, 28, 30, 81, 86
saddle fitting 86
saddles 83, 107
salt 44
seaweed 44
shod 57, 59, 61, 63, 78
shoeing 57
stabling 72
stress 34, 62

strip grazing 40, 70, 71
sweet orange 91
sycamore 52

tack 10, 22, 34, 73, 80, 81, 82, 83, 84, 86, 90, 92, 131, 133, 140, 141, 161
tack fitter 82
tea tree 89, 93
track system 67, 69, 70, 176, 179, 189
turmeric 43

ulcers 41, 49, 67, 173

vet 10, 16, 23, 24, 26, 28, 29, 31, 35, 38, 69, 76, 100, 101, 105, 112, 134, 135, 144, 151, 152, 161, 169, 173, 175
violet leaf 92
vitamins 42, 44, 45, 49

water 45
white clover 50

yew 53

zoopharmacognosy 88